SHADOW MAN

SHADOW MAN

A NOVEL

JEFFREY FLEISHMAN

STEERFORTH PRESS
HANOVER, NEW HAMPSHIRE

For information about permission to reproduce
selections from this book, write to:
Steerforth Press L.L.C., 45 Lyme Road, Suite 208,
Hanover, New Hampshire 03755

Library of Congress Cataloging-in-Publication Data
Fleishman, Jeffrey.
 Shadow man : a novel / by Jeffrey Fleishman.
   p. cm.
 ISBN 978-1-58642-198-4 (alk. paper)
 1. Alzheimer's disease--Fiction. I. Title.
 PS3606.L457S53 2012
 813'.6--dc23

                    2012003398

Book design by Peter Holm, Sterling Hill Productions

1 3 5 7 9 10 8 6 4 2

For my parents
ANNE AND TONY
and the memories they keep alive.

I remember him coming home from shipyards and factories, boots clicking and thumping down the sidewalk, and him whistling and smoking a rolled cigarette, metal flakes in his hair, hands stained and chipped as if he were wandering in from a war. Then into the kitchen for a gulp of beer; if it was summer, he'd step onto the back stoop and stare over rooftops of antennas to the gathering moon. The sky soothed him. Twilight was his time, not that he ever told me to stay away; it's just that sometimes you know when not to crowd a man. I watched him through the screen, setting my breaths to his and staying invisible, like a spy or a saint or a moth in the shadows.

I can't even recall yesterday and here I am tracing the edges of decades ago — I think it's been that long — in a Philly neighborhood of men standing on stoops and drinking Genny. They were statues, all of them, different shapes and sizes, yes, but statues all the same, with raised, cocked arms and tilted-back heads. Sips and slurps played into the night and crumpled cans clattered off the rims of garbage bins as women hurried suppers onto tables and boys like me crossed ourselves, bowed for grace, and counted our sins. What keeps drifting through me, though, like breeze off a sea, is that summer after Mom died, the same year Richard Nixon scowled sweaty and sinister and I started noticing newspaper headlines and halter tops. For some reason girls in halter tops stand out; bare shoulders and tanned backs moving in wondrous rhythms. It was the year my dad told me to call him Kurt.

He was painting navy ships. His days were creosote, endless cans of flat gray (You ever consider, Jim, how many goddamn cans of paint go on an aircraft carrier?), and the salt-egg-diesel-in-the-water-tang of the *Delaware* before she slipped her shoals and opened to the Atlantic. He'd get transfixed by oil slicks of purple, gold, and aluminum shimmying past him in the water like abstract paintings, pondering their molecular structures, deciphering maps and designs in the thread-lines of their intricate shapes. He'd come home exhausted. Our house smelled of Bengay and rubbing ointments and was scattered with bandages that seemed like shards and pieces of ghosts. Blackened jeans hung on doorknobs and white T-shirts, turned amber with sweat and streaked with gray and muddied red, were draped over the banister as if a man could shed himself, peeling to nakedness and standing in the shower, steam seeping through the second floor like fog.

That was Kurt five days a week, sometimes six if the foreman offered overtime, but never on Sunday. Kurt had a passion most guys who painted ships didn't: tennis. He loved it, especially the few times he played on grass, the skitter and slide of the ball, its unpredictability. Growing up, he didn't like football or baseball, so he'd head to the tennis court with its drooped net that looked like laundry shot up by a machine gun. He learned the game from an old guy who wore overalls and walked his dog around the playground. This old guy reveled in the game's mathematical complexities. He passed his tricks on to Kurt — the topspin, the slice backhand, the toss on the serve, the way to sneak in for a volley. "Creep in like an aberration," the old guy would say, rasping and huffing when he spoke.

Every US Open, he'd drive Kurt to Jake's Tavern and they'd sit studying the players like they were two rich guys at Flushing Meadows, the old guy breaking peanuts and drinking beer, Kurt sipping soda till he nearly exploded, the dog lying on the cool floor. The old guy's favorite saying was: "Hit the ball on the rise, that's where the magic lies." One day, the old guy didn't show up, and then didn't show up the next, either. Kurt had heard something happened to him, but it was vague, whispered. Kurt didn't want to know, really, so he let it go, gratified to have the can of balls and the racquet and a book of diagrams the old guy had left him. But he'd tell me later that he wondered about that old guy; said you can't forget a man who gives you something that's deep inside yourself to begin with. You're bound to him, probably through the ages.

On Sundays, Kurt would lose his workingman self. He'd get up early and go to his special drawer, the one holding his white tennis shorts, white shirt, and white wool socks. They were the only clothes he ever ironed and he'd get mad as hell if I so much as peeked in that drawer. He'd dress, tiptoe past my room, and head out the door on pale legs, walking up the burned-brick street, past the flats of his working buddies who teased him about being uppity, joking with him about wanting a "spot of tea," then he'd jump on the El and cross out of the city to neighborhoods with lawn sprinklers and tennis courts with no cracks. I went with him a few times. He was compact and graceful, flowing across the court like rain squiggling down a window. He was quick, too, hitting lines and angles, holding his power until needed. His serve curved and kicked in hard, and his backhand was a one-handed swoop of symmetrical perfection. He cussed under his breath when he missed a shot; an unforced error was a dreaded thing. Those rich guys from the suburbs didn't know what this scarred, rough painter of ships might do. But those times on the court were the only times I saw Kurt not as a father but as a man, a man who was part of me, yes, but one who had another dimension. I never asked him about it, but as I got older I understood there are parts that don't surrender to what the rest of you becomes. It is my experience that men have more of these parts than women, and that's what breaks them in the end, although I may be wrong. I have not studied it thoroughly.

The summer I called my dad Kurt was also known to Kurt and me as the summer of Vera. She burst into our neighborhood diner on a Friday night, one of those people you hear coming before you see them, not like the cowboys in the movies who ride in from way off in the distance without making a sound. Vera jangled. She plucked a menu from the slot near the silver cash register and pulled it to her eyes and ran her fingers across each line as if she were reading Dostoevsky or a lawn mower manual, something you had to pay real close attention to. Everyone looked up quick, got a glance, and then stared down at the Formica tops, counting those little gold flecks, hoping, praying this woman would pass them the way a storm skims in real close and then mysteriously whirls away. She spotted Kurt and me sitting by the window, minding our own business, trying to scrunch small, but you can't get too small in a window seat, especially at night when the lights outside put you on a kind of stage. She headed right for us. Kurt said under his breath: "Shit."

"You boys look lonely."

"No, we're pretty good," Kurt said.

"Well, you look lonely to me. What are your names? Mine's Vera, and I'm tired of driving. Exasperated, you might say. I saw this ragged-lit place from the road. You know Edward Hopper? This diner could have slipped off one of his canvases." She held up a spoon, polished it with a napkin. "I need some tea. Tea with lemon. I prefer it that way, although I know the Brits drink it with milk, but I never did trust the Brits, not since my first boyfriend, he was a Brit, ran off with a good friend, at the time it seemed she was, anyway. Scooch over and let me in."

Vera slid next to Kurt and kept chattering. Chatterers drove him insane, the same way unforced errors did. I was still trying to figure out Edward Hopper.

Vera's face was fury and delight. Soft yet angular, it was hardened by eyeliner and lipstick; a face you could kiss and fight with in a single moment. I decided she was pretty, especially in profile. Her voice, despite its chattiness, was husky, bruised almost, a late-night-movie voice kind of like Lizabeth Scott's, this old Hollywood actress with a slight lisp Kurt was in love with. Every Sunday when the *Inquirer* hit the doorstep, he'd grab the *TV Guide* and go through each day of the week hoping for a Lizabeth Scott movie. If he found one, a little hoot would echo through the house and he'd circle the time and channel, and if it wasn't too late, maybe a little past midnight, he'd haul me to the TV to watch it with him. I was more into Wonder Woman, but there was something alluring about Lizabeth Scott, luminous in black and white, like she was part of an ancient story that would keep playing even after the TV went off and the glow on the screen shrank to the size of a dime before going dark.

Vera kept talking and Kurt kept sliding in the booth and Vera kept sliding after him, until Kurt was pretty much pressed against the window. "I'm glad I met you two fine gentlemen," said Vera. "You live around here?"

"Up the street a ways. Not close, in fact it's kinda far, now that I think about it. It's pretty far, huh, Jim?"

"A good ways away."

"Well, Kurt, here's the deal. I need a place to stay. I'm in a little trouble."

"What kind?"

"The kind a woman gets into and can't easily get out of."

"That could be a lot of things."

"A man."

"What kind of man?"

"The worst damn kind."

"I don't know, Vera. Me and the boy stay to ourselves."

We were definitely in a Lizabeth Scott moment. Kurt knew it, too. It came over his face the way a mathematical equation suddenly makes sense to you. But Kurt was holding back, and Vera kept pressing. She ordered more tea and played with lemon slices like they were tiny suns setting in Kurt's periphery. Kurt kept his eyes straight ahead, sometimes looking at me to help him out, and I kept trying to think of something, but deep down I didn't mind if Vera came home with us. It had been a lonely house.

"This man," said Kurt, "is he big?"

"Not especially. But he's meaner than hell. He once shot two guys in the same day."

Kurt moved in his seat.

"Man, Kurt, you're easy. I'm teasing you. The guy's not big, but he's evil, sinister. Like a phantom."

It was hard to know if she was telling the truth.

"I don't want to know about it," Kurt said.

"Best not to."

Vera reached over and brushed the hair off my forehead with her fingers. It felt strange and nice, and she told me that I looked a little like Kurt, only handsomer, which made me smile, and I could see Kurt wanted to smile, too, but he stayed quiet by the window, thinking. Vera hummed "(I Can't Get No) Satisfaction" by the Rolling Stones and asked me if I wanted to dance, but I said no. I had never seen anyone dance in the diner, except when Billy Doyle played "Fly Me to the Moon" on the jukebox and danced with a bottle of Thunderbird and an imaginary girlfriend after he pitched a no-hitter in church-league softball. Vera hummed another tune and reached for Kurt's hand; no woman had touched that hand since Mom died.

"I need help," she said.

Kurt told me to go pay the check. I watched from the cash register as he leaned in and talked to Vera as if he were bargaining over the price of a stolen watch. I didn't know what he would do, but by the time I got back with the change, Kurt was standing by the booth, and in the next instant we were strolling out the door with Vera between us. She laced her arms into Kurt's and mine and said an adventure was beginning. It seemed surreal to be walking through

6

our neighborhood with this new person leaning warm against me. Surreal being a word I'd discovered along with luminous a few days earlier on my daily scan of the dictionary in which I had promised Mom to learn every English word before I died. I told this to Vera and she kept repeating "surreal," saying she liked the way it curled in her mouth and melted away.

We got to the house and opened the door and, suddenly, I felt Mom's presence. She was cool on my shoulder, the way nighttime air whistles through a window crack. She died the winter before the summer Dad said I could call him Kurt. She was making a cake and had run out of brown sugar so she hurried out of the house and down the street to Merle's Market, and as she was coming back, a Fleetwood skidded on ice, jumped onto the sidewalk, and killed her. A Fleetwood in our neighborhood meant a bookie or a mob-connected guy was tracking debts in the numbers racket. We never found out. No one saw the license plate, and the car sped away in a black flash through the snow. Mom had left the oven on preheat, flour on the table, and two egg yolks in a Pyrex mixing bowl. That scene was as precise as a still life, more vivid than her funeral mass or the way the sleet blew sideways when men my dad worked with burned the frost off the dirt and lowered Mom into the earth. I missed her; her linen dresses and her scent — Chanel and Clabber Girl Baking Soda — and her slacks and half shirts and her hair pulled back and bouncing. She would slide behind me, wrap me in her arms, and whisper in my ear, and sometimes she'd make me cut vegetables for dinner, laughing as onions made us both cry and joking until Dad (Kurt) got home and pulled out a beer, washed his face in the sink, and turned and hugged her, her back bending on his big forearms, telling him to get cleaned up better than that if he wanted to get kissed back, which he always did, but not before he stepped out on the stoop and breathed in the ending of the day. That's the pretty version and the one I'm sticking with, but to be honest, the real version was not that far off. We were happy.

Vera wasn't the kind of woman to be shy about taking another woman's space. She stepped across the threshold and told Kurt to put water on for tea and then she went upstairs and took a bath. She came down an hour later in one of Kurt's T-shirts and a pair of cutoffs and sat at the kitchen table as if she'd been living in that house since it was built. Kurt seemed mystified, too, and we looked at each other as if to say, *Who's going to tell her the rules?* but neither of us said a thing until Vera poked into the refrigerator and sighed."Kurt, where are the lemons?"

We never had lemons in the house, but Kurt said, "Hmmm. We must be out." Without another word, Vera grabbed her bulky macramé, fringe-swinging purse and disappeared out the door. Kurt looked at me and said: "I don't know if I like her or not, but she is direct." Unabashed, I thought, and went to the dictionary.

Vera came back with lemons, oranges, and grapefruits and squeezed them all into a pitcher and shoved it in the freezer and started talking about Cairo and the pyramids and the Nile and about these guys called muezzins who sing prayers from minarets shaped like flutes and how on a feast called Eid they slaughter sheep across the city, blood flowing in the streets and alleys and everyone giving thanks to Allah and feeding the poor.

"How do you know all this?" said Kurt.

"I was there, honey."

"In Cairo?"

"All across the Delta."

I thought Kurt was going to say Mississippi, but he thought better of it. Vera and her friends had hiked across North Africa years ago, starting in Cairo then to Alexandria and then into Libya, Tunisia, Algeria, and Morocco. She spoke of Bedouins and fires in the desert and storms that blew through the sand. She kept talking as if the whole trip were playing out in front of her, every detail an ornate creation, much better and more alive than the slide shows we had at school and those *National Geographic* pictures that were beautiful but seemed too pretty to be real. Vera's stories were ragged and exotic and full of things like horses galloping along beaches or the sounds of hammered copper, and big bazaars, and a souk in Marrakesh, where a man with skin the color of eggplant and eyes like blue ice reached his hand into a sack of saffron and held it up like gold. Marrakesh, what a word. Three syllables of music. Mar-ra-kesh. I think I heard it once in a Lizabeth Scott movie, or maybe it was a film with Humphrey Bogart, whom Kurt wasn't crazy about, but I found him believable in most roles. Marrakesh. Tripoli. Carthage. Vera was lucky, and I felt lucky, too, just listening. I looked over at Kurt, and he was following Vera's stories. She was chattering, yes, but Kurt was enthralled and every now and then he looked for a spot to interject something. He'd fill with air, but then he'd hold it as if wondering how a guy who paints ships in Philly can spin out something as remarkable as Marrakesh. But finally, after Vera had trekked us across the Maghreb — I had to look that one up — Kurt couldn't hold it in any longer.

"I play tennis on grass," he said.

A pause. A too-long pause.

Vera laughed and reached out for Kurt's hand. He pulled it back, not fast or startling but in a way a plate is cleared from a table. Vera laughed again, but she clipped it. Kurt smiled one of his famous half smiles that kept you guessing, and I think Vera caught this, too. The conversation changed to things more American, closer to home and graspable (a word that looks funny but does exist), but I thought Vera had a lot more desert stories in her and I hoped to hear them all.

The light was warm over the kitchen table. A sixty-watt yellow glow that obscured the exactness of things not directly in the light; they lingered in the shadowy edges the way actors stand in the wings before a cue leads them into the floodlights. I could hear rain falling in the alleys. It rattled over our stoop and set the neighborhood dogs running. They barked close and then distant and then I heard children sloshing near the manhole covers that bubble up when it storms. Lightning flashed, but there wasn't much thunder and soon the storm passed, leaving soaked kids and a coolness behind. I left Kurt and Vera in the kitchen and walked down the alley to St. Jude's. The streets were slick and pure, black mirrors reflecting the gray ghosts of clouds racing overhead in the wind and, every now and then, a break in the clouds and a glimmer of moon. The rain had cleaned the dust from the church's stained-glass windows; I studied the deep, rich colors of the saints, the artistry of their beards and hands and their eyes, the way they followed you, watching you from up there, frozen, but at night, after a rain, they seemed alive. I walked to the front of the church; water poured from the drain spouts and made mud beneath the holly bushes. The stairs were slippery, the railings rusty.

Father Heaney's head was bowed in the rectory window. He was likely reading one of his mystery novels. He once told Kurt they cleared his head after tending the sick and hearing confessions littered with "misdemeanors and a few felonies from the unexpected." Russet-haired with a pink Irish face, Fr. Heaney had given me my first communion years earlier. There is a lot to think about in that second when Jesus hovers before you, crisp and hard and then softening on your tongue and melting into you and becoming part of you in a slow dissolve as you cross yourself and walk back to your pew, tasting cardboard and grain, but knowing it's Jesus who rose from the dead to save your soul. I like that moment of believing. Fr. Heaney told Kurt — he was always pulling Kurt aside after Saturday-evening mass — that the act of communion was "transcendence of the spirit." Transcendence was one of my first dictionary words. Transcendence will lead you through the dictionary, which is really a book of clues, to spirit, revelation, and redemption. The only problem with communion was that you had to go to confession first, whisper your sins through a web of cheesecloth to the silhouette of Fr. Heaney, who knew who you were no matter how hard you tried to disguise your voice. Once I tried a Peter Lorre imitation and Fr. Heaney laughed and said: "Jim, just give it to me straight." I didn't tell him all my sins. Some of them belonged to me and not to God.

I was going to knock, but I left Fr. Heaney alone with his mystery novel. The city was quiet, its great energy washed and calmed by the rain. Dogs were rooting in the garbage of a blown-over trash can, and I walked home and stepped up the stoop and into the kitchen. Kurt and Vera were drinking vodka and lemonade, sitting across from each other like two poker players; Kurt cagey and Vera garrulous, making you wonder if she had a full house or a handful of nothing. They weren't drunk but they were happy.

"When you hit a backhand, Vera, your body flows in one long twist. People think a forehand is easier to hit than a backhand, but I disagree. A backhand is more natural, and much prettier when hit correctly. It's like opening up your wings to fly."

Forty-six words. Kurt had spoken forty-six words. A paragraph. Without stopping. It might have been a record.

"Teach me to hit a backhand, Kurt."

"One day, maybe."

"Now."

"It's dark and there's no court."

"In the alley."

Tennis was sacred to Kurt, and Vera was asking him to hit in the alley, which I suspected may have been sacrilege. Kurt sat for a minute. He sipped his lemonade and vodka. He got up and left the room, and I figured this was the end of Vera. But Kurt returned with a tennis racquet (not his best one) and two cans of balls (old). He walked into the alley.

"Jim, get down there. Vera, come here."

He gave her the racquet. She slipped between his arms. Kurt bent her body and taught her the flow of the backhand. Vera hit wet balls down the alley. I chased them and threw them back. She was laughing and Kurt was telling her to concentrate and to pretend she was lifting into flight. One time she did and the ball zipped down the alley with topspin, water streaming off it like a shooting star in a telescope. I ran after it into the dark, my breath and heart beating harder, my sneakers soaked, a smile breaking across my face. The whole neighborhood was sleeping except the three of us and when I turned with the soggy ball in my hand, Kurt and Vera shimmered like cutouts in the night. As I walked closer, I heard their voices and for a moment pretended that Mom was home and nothing had changed. Another rainstorm rolled in and Vera and I went running for the house while Kurt jumped on the stoop and back off again, juggling two balls in puddles beneath the sputtering streetlight like some crazy kid or a guy with a night pass to the carnival.

There's light through the window shade. It's morning, or perhaps some luminary trick. I'm lying on my back like a corpse, waiting for what, I don't know. I think something's supposed to happen. It seems to me there should be sounds by now, some shape moving toward me. I try to remember my name. I can't, but I know I am somebody; I can count my fingers. Is every day like this? I don't know. I know Kurt and Vera by heart. They live inside of me, and I know that they were real. I can still hear them. The shade is bright with light and someone, a woman in white, is saying, "Good morning, James." I must be James because she's pulling down my sheet and propping me up on a pillow. She hands me a glass of water. It seems like this scene has happened a million times, but I can't recall what happens next. The woman in white opens a drawer and rattles things; she combs my hair and holds a mirror up. An old man looks back. Not old, entirely. Maybe fifty or fifty-two. Lines fan out from the eyes, but the face is sharp, perhaps a bit slack under the chin. The hair is gray and black, the color of a sweater Kurt used to wear, but Kurt's is not the face I'm looking at, although there is a resemblance. The man in the mirror, not a bad-looking guy really, seems lost, as if he's trying to remember where he put the car keys, or how he ended up at the bank when he was aiming for the grocery store. I look at the woman in white. Then to the mirror. "That's you, James. Hurry up, we've got to get you ready. Eva is coming today." I can't recall who Eva might be, maybe another woman in white. Flowers sit in a vase on a table near the bed, and there's a little desk in the corner under the window. The desk is covered in papers and books. "Are you going to write today, James?" I don't know. Is that what I do? The woman in white pours me juice and hands me a pill. I seem to know what to do, so this must have happened a million times, although if it did, the woman in white should know I prefer grapefruit juice to orange juice. Prefer comes from preferential. The woman in white pulls up the shade, and for a moment she disappears in the light that rushes into the room. "A new day, James." I guess it is.

"Where am I?"

"You're where you've been for the last two years. St. Jude's home."

"Is this heaven?"

The woman in white laughs as if I've made a joke, but I feel completely serious.

"No, James, this is earth."

"What city?"

"Philadelphia."

"Philadelphia."

"You were born here, not far from where you're sitting right now, if you look out that window across the rooftops and the steeples. There's not as many steeples as there used to be, with churches moving out to the suburbs and leaving us in a city without God."

"God is a concept by which we measure our pain. John Lennon said that."

"Well, I don't know about John Lennon, but seems like a little of that memory of yours is kicking in. Might be one of the good days."

"John Lennon was a Beatle. The best one in my opinion, although Paul had a gift for melody. The others I can't remember. Who's Eva?"

"You know who Eva is, James. Think."

The woman in white lays out my clothes on the bed as if I'm a child. Khakis, a blue buttondown shirt, gray socks, a brown braided belt. She says I need a shave and leads me to the bathroom and sets me in front of the big mirror over the sink. She runs the water, hands

14

me a razor and a can of shaving cream. She leans against the wall and watches. I have two thoughts: Why am I here? And if I know what to do with a razor and shaving cream, why can't I remember this lady Eva who is coming to visit me? The razor scrapes. It's a sound I know well, a soft sound, like sand on waxed paper. Every shave peels away a mask and brings a new man. I seem to know this analogy; maybe it's from Kurt, maybe from those times when I was a boy standing in the bathroom watching him the way this woman in white is watching me. It's a nice thought, to be new. I finish shaving and am pointed toward the shower. The woman in white steps outside the door, but leaves it open a crack. The water runs hard and warm; it feels good, washing away the clenched feeling the face has after a shave. I dry and put on my clothes. The bed is made and I sit on it. I smell of powder and deodorant. The vase on the table holds flowers; they look fresh.

A man, a doctor, slips into the room and asks me questions and writes things on a clipboard. He says I have a far-back but not close memory; my childhood vivid, my adulthood dormant, colorless. What I see, witness, experience one day disappears the next, like that shiny plastic paper I wrote on as a kid; when you lifted the paper off the inky board, whatever you had drawn was gone so you could begin anew. There are, apparently, endless analogies for what's happening to my shriveling mind. A small part of my brain resembles a glacier with deep recesses sunlight cannot penetrate. He says it's like when ice climbers descend into a fissure and the light dims as they dangle on ropes in the darkness. The doctor says there will be fewer fissures of light, and eventually all will be black, except for an occasional flash of unexplained lightning that may revive a memory for a few seconds or maybe an hour, but it doesn't matter because it won't last and the memory won't be remembered anyway. Confetti in the wind; a shattered mosaic; these are other examples he uses. He brims with metaphor. The doctor is heavyset with a broad face and curly brown hair that glows in the window light. He speaks quietly but in a determined, uninterrupted flow, like a book on tape, or a man telling you interesting facts between train stops. He is intrigued by me or, more precisely, my case; I am younger than the ashen-faced droolers lingering in hallways of piss and peppermint and that antiseptic scent that makes the floors sticky. That's what excites him, my youth. I am, he says, very young "for such depletion." Usually, a mind in my state is seventy or seventy-five years old, but I have somehow "depleted" earlier and this concerns the doctor, who says it's happening more and more as baby boomers age; a whole generation dangling in the dark. He says he suspects "environmental causes mixed with the stresses of modern life that somehow, in its technology, has done something to the mind." He speaks of synapses, brain circuitry, and promising drugs that have done wonders with rats. I have a headache. I want to ask him a question but I don't. I just sit in my powder smell, staring at the flowers until he leaves. What is there to say about lost ice climbers?

"Do you want one of your books on photography, James? You like those."

Does the woman in white ever go home, I wonder.

I shake my head and she leaves the room. I go to the table. It's messy with *Philadelphia Inquirer*s, books (Emerson, Updike, Edward Weston), pens (Uni-balls), and notebooks scrawled with pictures, words, and stray, strange symbols. On one page "James" is written one thousand times in minuscule letters as if with a rat's paw. On other pages paragraphs seem to lift out of nowhere as if they arrived uninvited, without context. One notebook is full of stories copied exactly from the *Inquirer*, except for the bylines, which all read "James." I am James. I write the name James; the penmanship is the same. These are my notebooks. There's a box on the table. I open it. There's a stack of newspaper clippings inside, most from the *Los Angeles Times*. I pull the top one out. It's dated September 12, 2001. The headline reads

TERRORISTS ATTACK NEW YORK, PENTAGON. Fireballs and huge blossoms of smoke roll out of two buildings that look like silver pillars in a war without soldiers. Under the picture there's a story written by James Ryan. There's that name James again. I pull other clippings from the box. They are all written by James Ryan; some go back twenty years. I am James Ryan. I write for newspapers. Do I still? If this is me I've been to Prague and Budapest, Baghdad and Tehran, and many other places I don't remember. But these are documents and datelines; they don't lie, don't appear mysteriously out of folders; no, they are real. There are pictures with the stories. One is of a crowd in the snow, stony faces peeking through a gray dusk dotted with ripped umbrellas, raised gloved fists, and a husky man with a full mustache and a bullhorn suspended above the crowd, transfixed in twilight, his eyes like dark fire. The caption identifies the man as Lech Walesa. I know that name, but I don't; who is that name? I stare at the face, run my fingers over it, but he is meaningless to me, a stranger.

Another picture shows bearded men in the desert, bandoliers crisscrossing their chests, their faces hard and thin, their white teeth flashing, all of them standing in the back of a pockmarked pickup truck. They seem a ragged army of bank robbers or castaway nomads in the desert. The caption says they are mujahideen fighting American forces in a place called Anbar. I study their faces, too. But nothing comes. How can it not come? My name is there in ink. James Ryan. James Ryan was in Anbar with wild, bearded men. How does one forget that?

My head hurts. I close the box. I pick up another notebook. Pages and pages filled with spirals drawn in red, black, and blue ink; they look like twisters and tornadoes, storms whirling across paper. Another notebook is full of noses. Drawings and drawings of noses, fat, slim, long, bulbous, pert noses. They remind me of when I was a boy with Kurt and we went to a Halloween store to try on masks and I picked out a big waxy nose attached to black glasses and bushy eyebrows. Kurt said I looked like Jerry Lewis in *The Nutty Professor*. Why can I remember Jerry Lewis and not Budapest?

I pick up the Emerson book and sit on my bed. I don't read it. I hold its worn hard cover and let the sunlight warm me. I see steeples out the window, crosses pricking the sky, sneakers draped over phone lines. It seems familiar to me, as if out there on those streets part of me wanders. I step closer to the window. I am suspended over the city. I see a bridge, a twist of river, row houses, pigeons, laundry on rooftops, a silver train silent in the distance, racing beyond the car traffic and out of sight, so sleek and beautiful. There's a park to the left. The leaves are yellow, plum, and brown. It must be the last days of autumn; I imagine I can hear the fallen leaves scratching the street, spinning in crinkly coils in the alleys. I try to go back to that last image, but it's gone; my thoughts are ether, burning one brilliant moment and then vanishing. Perhaps they return, but how can I know.

I hear shoes squeaking. I turn from the window and see a woman in white. She smiles and steps into the room. There is someone behind her. The woman in white smiles, turns, and leaves the room. The lady standing near the window with me has dark hair, black, I think, but I can't say for sure — sunlight plays tricks with color. Her face is sharp and pale, not sickly pale, but radiant, as if lit from inside. Her eyes are aluminum blue; her lipstick is red, but a quiet red; her hands are the long hands of a magician, or maybe a seamstress or a sculptor. She reaches into her purse and pulls out a paper scribbled with ink. She unfolds it; it makes no sound. She looks at me, then at the paper. She reads:

> *The world is changing around us. The tanks, the placards, the snow and winter's bite, a revolution moving like a ripple through water. I love you. I love this hotel. Outside, the streets are finally quiet. It is nearly dawn. The last protestor*

*is clopping home. You sleep in your clothes; I carve you
from the darkness. I write another story. Can you hear the
keystrokes? Dawn is an hour or two away, and soon we'll be
off again into history . . .*

She folds the paper and slides it back into her purse. She puts her
hands on my face, her thumbs skimming gently beneath my eyes.
Her perfume I do not know. She looks hard into my eyes, studies
them, as if something is written on them, a language or thoughts to
decipher. Her hands slide from my face, brush my shoulders, and
withdraw. I look at her, maybe the way a man looks at a map from
another country. She sighs.

"You don't remember that, do you? You wrote those words in
1989. In Prague, after Havel led them through the streets. James,
you must remember. They are your words, in your hand, to me. I
was the one sleeping in my clothes in the night. Don't you remember
how we laughed about working so hard that we slept in our clothes
and woke up wrinkled."

She steps closer and whispers into my ear.

"Sometimes we slept without our clothes. You must remember,
James, the snow falling outside. Who am I, James?"

I want to know who she is, but I do not.

"I am Eva. The girl you met when the world changed."

three

I am the woman in white.

He doesn't know my name; doesn't remember my face. Every day he asks: "Are you the woman in white from yesterday? I think there was one yesterday." I listen to Eva tell him those stories; what a time it must have been, on the brink of so much. How can he not know this? He is young and handsome, the way men get when they start to gray, an angular classicism. His mind shouldn't be so decrepit. These other drones in here, okay, they've slipped away. I see them, blank and ghost-eyed, fortunate their bodies move to permutations other than thought. Or is it? I don't know. But he is younger and should not be so lost.

He tells me every day about Kurt and Vera. They're the only alive things in that brain of his. I listen and imagine as he repeats their story under his breath. I am good at that. As a child I played make-believe, running through hidden passageways and lurking beneath windows, spying on neighbors with pocket cameras and decoder rings. Life is best understood in whispers, not in laughter and loud voices; we carry with us the secret things that quietly wear us away. I watched birds, too. My binoculars scanned the skies over fields of wildflowers and thistle. Dusk was the best time to see them, flying against the invading darkness; swift birds with tiny hearts and wings of purple, yellow, and black, and higher, hawks circling on wind currents like kings and queens in a storybook. I collected fallen feathers and taped them to my closet door, which over the years grew into a plume as lush as a Cherokee headdress. Birds were magic to me. They could go anywhere. I was a gangly girl, untamed knees and elbows peeking from my communion dress, lost in the silk and taffeta of my prom gown. I evened out eventually and, although I am not a beauty, men have suggested I possess a bookish sexiness. I can never tell if that is a promise or a lie. There is so little space between the two, and as any woman knows men are capable of the sweetest phrases between happy hour and last call. I suppose it means I am thin and wear glasses and tied-back hair but have good breasts and clear skin. Even in adolescence, when other girls cotton-balled themselves with astringents and emollients, my skin was as bright as an empty page. James doesn't mention such things. He offers no compliments, tells no half-truths; he looks at me the way a stranger does in a grocery store, a flicker of recognition that vanishes as the carts pass. I hope for more. The doctors, the administration, no one knows the secret bond I have to James. The way I appeared — an applicant with strong recommendations seeking work in an institution with high turnover — is a matter of perseverance with which I have been blessed. A natural talent, I suppose, in the way a handyman is gifted to fix broken blenders and sewing machines. We each have our proclivities, those things big and small that make us unique and enviable in the eyes of others. I suspect I am not much envied, although I do have, despite my previously mentioned active imagination, a reputation for pragmatism, but that may be the twin of perseverance. I prefer to think of myself as a quiet multitude of unappreciated qualities.

If that sounds bitter, I am not. I am a woman searching amid hallways, carrying syringes and paper cups of pills. I like the weight of the stethoscope around my neck, and sometimes I listen to my heart, marveling at the mystery of its energy and wondering how and when it will stop. Tick-tock. I don't linger on such thoughts. I have a mission. I carry James's chart. It is battered and heavy, and although I write neatly in it, meticulous in my numbers and abbreviations, it is filled with pages of what we nurses call "doctor-scratch." I cannot read it all but I know what it says about advancing Alzheimer's, the shutdown of the light field across the medial temporal lobes (MTL), where the larva-shaped hippocampus loses its grasp of memory, perhaps caused long ago by trauma or maybe a disfigured gene or other predisposition that lurked in the tissue since birth only to one day bloom with mischievous intent. There are so many ways for a mind to tumble and lose itself in worlds far from us. The body on those Discovery Channel documentaries is glorious, intricate, and strong, a wonder of God conspiring with nature, but really we are as fragile as rice paper, ruined over time by imperceptible rips and tears.

I search for clues on a color-coded poster of the brain in profile I kept from nursing school. It strikes me that the most ingenious thing about us humans — not counting the soul — looks like a boxing glove. Atop which, to borrow a metaphor from James's curly haired doctor, the cerebral cortex hovers like a trapped cloud. Where are the answers? I study the science and anatomy of James, his blood pressure, reflexes, temperature, the dose of his cholinesterase inhibitors, but I don't know him, not even on my late shift, when all the doctors are home and I hold his CAT scans to the light and he floats before me, fleshless, a silver-gray apparition, yielding little. His hip bones resemble folded wings, his forearms flutes, his legs strange spindly reeds. He has five fillings, a broken rib that must have been untended when he was a boy, healing poorly, leaving the thread of disjointed marrow. This is what the pictures of science and technology bare. This is what I see. It is not enough. I need him to come back.

four

The marshlands south of Philly stretch to Wilmington and to beaches beyond; they glisten brown and green in the wind and make you think of another time. We skated by them in Kurt's Impala, the windows down, our hair flying and me wedged between Vera and Kurt in the front seat. The radio played so loud that it was a cacophony (I had my dictionary on the trip) of static and breeze, although every now and then a recognizable tune burst through, like the guitar lick in "Signs" by the Five Man Electrical Band or the chords of the great wa-wa opening of Black Sabbath's "Iron Man."

We came around a bend and drove over a small bridge, the Impala bouncing along as if racing across a surface made of stretched rubber bands. I thought I heard "Tiny Dancer," and when I looked over I swore Vera was mouthing the words, but I couldn't be sure because her hair was a black sea tossing around her. Kurt stopped for coffee at a shack with a sandy parking lot. Vera got out and pointed her face toward the sun, leaning on the car and asking Kurt to buy her lemons. Kurt walked through a screen door and flies scattered and I saw an old black man with a tilted hat peek up from behind the counter as if he had been awakened; he smiled the colors of stained ivory and broken gold.

"I love a car trip, don't you, Jim?"

"Sometimes they get too long."

"Can you read a map?"

"Not too well."

"Unfolding them is like opening a mystery. New worlds stretching before you in circuitous lines. There's a word for you, Jim. Circuitous.

You can run your fingers along roads and mountains and coasts. I wish I'd have lived centuries ago. I would have been an explorer. But you know something? I'm tired after a car trip. I think that's funny, don't you? You're just sitting for hours, listening to music and wind, but it takes it out of you, you know? Maybe, it's the sun, and the distance, and your body having to re-gather in a new place."

I looked out the window to Vera. She had on shorts and a white halter top with a collar and black buttons on the front. She pulled back her hair and tied it with ribbon. I still couldn't tell how old she was. She was hard to read that way; she could be young, like that night a week or so ago when she was hitting tennis balls in the alley, or she could be older, like now with the sun and no shadows on her face. I heard the flat rubber sounds of cars passing in the distance and the bark of a boat horn coming from the ocean beyond the marshes. Kurt came out and handed me a Sprite and gave Vera a knife and a bag of lemons. Kurt sat on the hood, sipping his coffee, and Vera cut lemons, squeezing the juice in her mouth and not even wincing like most people do.

"Juiciest lemon I ever had was in Sorrento."

Kurt and I looked at each other.

"That's in Italy, boys, below Naples. The cliffs are high and the lemons are big as a grapefruit. You could fill a whole glass with one lemon. I swam in the blue sea and dreamed of sirens tempting sailors. Imagine voices so pretty that they lead you to ruin. Haunting. There's another word for you, Jim. Haunting. A voice out there in the mist, calling."

Kurt and I had seen *Jason and the Argonauts* on TV, but neither of us said anything and Vera went on slicing and squeezing lemons, the juice dripping down her forearms and elbows and into the sand. She could do that. Begin a story, frame it out pretty so as to invite you in, and then let it trail off the way a breeze lifts out of nowhere and vanishes.

Kurt tossed his coffee cup and we were off again. Marvin Gaye was on the radio, but we lost him when Kurt accelerated and the car filled with crackle and wind and Vera's flying hair. The road beyond the windshield was wide and not too curvy. Kurt was sweating and daydreaming, his hand loose on the wheel. What was going on? It wasn't like Kurt to take a vacation so suddenly. He hadn't been off work since Mom died, but the summer days and Vera enticed him. We still didn't know her real story, or at least I didn't. Kurt may have because he and Vera had been staying up long nights talking. They weren't sleeping together. When I'd come down in the mornings, Kurt was back-flat on the floor and Vera was curled on the couch. They'd ease into the day like two cats; Kurt making coffee and pouring juice; Vera snatching the *Inky* from the porch, thumbing through pages and glancing at ads and pictures with the occasional, "Hey, Kurt look at this." Her clothes tangled with his, hanging off the banister and on the towel racks in the bathroom scented with her balms of lilac and musk. She'd sit on the back stoop and murmur Buddhist chants and sometimes it seemed she went into a trance. Neighbors peeked from behind window shades and Kurt told the Kowalskys and McMurphys that Vera was a "distant relative who had spent her life in exotic places." Vera played along, calling Kurt "Cuz" and inventing family histories.

She'd come into my room and lie beside me while I studied the dictionary, asking me to read her the second and third meanings of words. I'd read slow and I could feel my voice calm her or maybe it was the glow of the lamp and the sounds of distant cars in the alleys. She'd close her eyes and tell me that words were masks and disguises. "Did you know, Jim, that God has ninety-nine names in Arabic? The Avenger. The Truth. The Shaper of Beauty. They're written in holy books and on fortress walls deep in the desert. Go see these places one day, Jim. Promise me you'll go and trace God's name on a desert wall." A few times at night, while Kurt was sleeping,

I'd sneak and sit on the stairs and see Vera in her underpants and T-shirt kneeling beside the radiator, twirling her hair and staring at the front door as if waiting for someone to turn the knob. Once, I thought I heard her crying and talking to herself in the basement, and when she came up, wiping a startled look off her face, she told me she had been singing a rhyme from childhood and was sad that childhood would never come again. She put a picture of a yogi, a guy with a long beard who looked like he had diapers on and hadn't eaten in a while, on the coffee table. She bought beads and hung them between the kitchen and the dining room and then tried to teach Kurt to meditate by closing his eyes and sitting pretzel-legged, but Kurt cracked up and shook his head when she lit incense around him.

"Vera, this isn't me."

"You need to get in touch with your inner self."

"My inner self is doing just fine without me going to look for it."

Sprawling as she was in moods and scented possessions, though, Vera could not make the house her own, not even by carving her initials above the stove near the crucifix. Mom's spirit was there, not ready to give its blessing for Kurt to start a new life. That was fair. No one wants to be forgotten, especially in a house that held your pots and recipes and two boxes of stuff Kurt and I taped and wrote on with Magic Marker and slid into the attic next to the Christmas ornaments and a bicycle that had been there since before we moved in. It's hard to choose what you want to save of a person; it makes you wonder if you really knew them at all. Every scrap, shred, picture, scribbled note, favorite sweater is sacred.

Vera slipped in amid these things when we weren't looking. She brought stories that made the world bigger and more interesting. Our row house didn't have enough rooms to hold Vera's tales and Mom's memory, so Kurt, finding a streak of spontaneity I had only seen on the tennis court, stepped into my room just before dawn and announced: "Jim, we're hitting the road. Get dressed." He loaded us into the Impala when the streets were dewy and cool, and paperboys strained against their canvas sacks of headlines, while milkmen delivered bottles from Kensington to Fish Town to Rittenhouse Square. Paperboys and milkmen didn't need maps. They knew the alleys, back alleys, crevices, the fires in the drums near the trestles, the shantytowns on the riverbank and the iron and cement underbelly that kept the city from sinking. A lot of paperboys I knew were also altar boys; milkmen were pretty much just milkmen, except for Eddie Blankenridge who strangled widows in their bathrobes before the police arrested him climbing out of a window.

I had packed shorts, T-shirts, one pair of jeans, my dictionary, and the Beatles' *White Album*. You never know when you might come across a stereo. The *White Album* was my favorite, a jumble of moods and images. That's what I liked most about the Beatles; they were magpies (one of my favorite words, looked up after I heard it in a poem) gathering a little of this and a little of that and turning them into "Rocky Raccoon," "Cry Baby Cry," and "Savory Truffle." Vera liked the Beatles, too, but was more partial to the Rolling Stones and Tim Buckley. Kurt liked some guy named Walter Jackson, who had a deep, welling voice with no cracks, like a perfect sphere. That's all we had to listen to in the Impala — the radio and one Walter Jackson eight-track that kept sticking on song three until Kurt whacked it and it warbled back to the baritone of a man broken by the cruelty of love.

"Kurt, you have to buy more music."

"I could listen to Walter Jackson every hour of every day."

"I don't know if Jim and I can."

Kurt hit the gas and the car gripped the road, speeding south along the Delaware coast. Vera tried to light a cigarette but matches died against the wind. She cupped her hands and dipped her head below the glove box, and finally asked Kurt to slow down, which made

Walter Jackson louder, like God coming through a silver speaker. Vera took a drag and Kurt was off again, Vera's ember burning orange and fast. I kept looking over at her. Who was this woman? She said in the diner that night we met her that she was hiding from a man, and then with her stories of Cairo and Marrakesh I thought of her as a spy or a damsel of intrigue, an updated Lizabeth Scott with purple-tinted sunglasses and fingernails dotted with stars. Kurt wasn't telling me all he knew, and he seemed a different person, too, a man with more sides than I had once known. If I held him to the light I'd see all kinds of angles and colors. He started wearing sandals and skipped his normal haircut day at Johnny's; he didn't even shave every day, and on the days he didn't he looked like, but not exactly like, an apostle.

We crossed out of Delaware to Maryland and into eastern Virginia and the scents of bay crabs and marshes and smoked ham; signs for fireworks and summer squash. Moss hung in streaks and tresses, and the air was heavy. Dragonflies at the road's edge hovered over Queen Anne's lace and black-eyed Susies and buzzed away, slowly, as if flying through a sky of invisible honey. The earth was wild here, shaggy and vine-filled, devouring almost, yet serene, and the air clung to you like scrims of wet breath blowing across your shoulders and neck. Steeples slumped like tilted hats on wooden churches and rusted corrugated sheds, covered in strangling vines, sheltered lawn mowers and half-put-together motorcycles. Two men were gliding scythes through weeds and I swore I could hear their blades, the faintest rip and a whoosh of air, as if you ran your fingers through a cave of spider webs. They kept slicing like they were slow-dancing with crescents in the cool cut grass of a shade tree, their perimeter widening into the sun, but in no particular hurry. I could smell the grass. As we came around a bend, a black boy riding the whitest horse I had ever seen galloped through the thin pines, kicking up sand and needles and disappearing over a small bridge into the thicker woods. The boy had no saddle and he gripped the mane, flying almost, it seemed to me, his weight insubstantial and no burden on the muscle and bone moving beneath him. Vera spotted the boy. She turned her head as the car passed, watching the white horse shift from sunlight and shadow as it sprinted deeper into the woods toward another break of field, and maybe she was thinking of the Maghreb or some other distant place.

"I need to play tennis," Kurt announced.

He pulled the Impala over at a brick school off Route 13. There were two courts of cracked asphalt and ripped nets. Kurt looked at them and wondered if we should just move on, but he opened the trunk, pulled off his jeans, put on his tennis shorts, grabbed his Slazenger racquet and two cans of tennis balls. Vera put sun lotion on her face and lounged on the hood. Kurt started serving to an empty court and as he got to the fifth ball — before I could join him — a guy with spider crab legs and falling-down tube socks walked to the baseline with a racquet. He had an Afro and wore a tank top and sneakers ripped near the toes.

"You wanna hit?" he said in a drawl that seemed to mimic the way he sauntered along the fence.

"Why not?"

Kurt looked at me and winked. He started off easy, loping the ball deep toward the guy, settling into a rhythm. The guy struggled at first, misjudging balls, reacting too late, swinging wildly. But after a few minutes he settled and tugged his body tight, finding an economy of motion. Every move was a burst of concise energy, nothing wasted; it flowed through the shoulder to the elbow down the forearm through the wrist — a motion of flipping pancakes, only faster, tighter — to the sweet spot in the racquet, where the ball struck a clear chord, like a bass tuned to perfection or the voice of Walter Jackson. The guy was moving Kurt, pulling him with angles and variations of spin and speed, and Kurt was mixing it up with drop shots, slices, and down-the-line backhands, trying to crack the guy, but the guy was like a fish, darting when necessary and then rippling soft in a current. He was pretty to watch. Beads of sweat spattered around him on the baseline and evaporated in the sun. Kurt kept trying to find the guy's weak spot, but on some days, with some guys, there is no weak spot and Kurt lost two close sets. Kurt shook the guy's hand at the net and the two walked off the court; Kurt not minding, not too much anyway, being beat by a better player, a raggedly dressed guy out of the piney woods, and then saying how tennis was good that way, bringing strangers together, forcing them to share intimacies, showing themselves and their characters on the shots they chose.

Vera was sitting on the hood of the car, crying. She told Kurt and the guy that she loved watching the struggle between them; she said there was beauty in it and she slid off the hood and hugged Kurt and the guy and told them that out there on that old court with nobody around and the wind blowing hot through the trees two men came together and made magic. She said imagine how often that happens every day around the world, and nobody knows about it. Little scenes of magic played out in hidden places, witnessed only by a few and then tucked into the deep, deep memory of the world. She wiped her eyes and started laughing, embarrassed I guess, but I knew what she meant. Vera had a way of saying something you felt yourself. The guy stood talking for a while. He lived a mile to the east on tobacco land that had been sold off long ago and now grew cauliflower, which he and his family planted and harvested, except in the off-season and through the winter when they swept blood from the floor of the chicken factory, which, the guy said, gave off a scent that seemed to live in his nose hours after he went home and washed up.

"That smell is who we all are," said the guy. "My preacher, he works there, too, says it's the raw element of this world, connecting us all, animal and man alike, until God takes our souls."

"How long has your family been here?" said Vera.

"Since the ships came from Africa."

"You ever been?"

"To Africa? No. I ain't even been, I'll bet, more'n fifty miles from where I'm standing right now. Got no need. The world comes to us here, like you people. Taking Route 13 to that big bay bridge tunnel yonder. All I ever need to see of the world I can see through the windshields of passing cars."

"You play a lot of tennis?" said Kurt.

"See that school wall? I hit against it two hours a day. That wall is tougher than any man who ever played. The ball just keeps coming back, coming back. There's no time to think."

"Instinctive," said Kurt.

"If that's what you want to call it."

Kurt pulled a roll of grip tape from his bag and handed it to the guy. The guy thanked him and said good-bye; he walked past the edge of the court and toward the pines, his racquet spinning in his hand like a propeller.

"You believe in God, Jim?"

"I do."

"Kurt?"

"Mostly."

Vera sat back on the hood of the Impala and we were quiet. Kurt wiped sweat from his face. Tranquility is how my dictionary described it. Then the cicadas started a boisterous music in the trees, and that riled other noises, dragonflies dancing and bobbing over the car, Vera's rattling map, Kurt packing his tennis gear and sitting in the front seat, clicking the ignition, the eight-track squeaking to life and Walter Jackson rolling in like a storm from a great distance. We were off again, bound farther south toward the marshes that fringed the Chesapeake Bay Bridge Tunnel, the tang of egg, wet, and reed filling the air, salty on our tongues and slipping into our lungs. Egrets and smaller white and gray birds took flight around us, keeping pace with the Impala and then peeling off in silent arcs while above the windshield and over the water gulls glided on the crosswinds, their wings outstretched and still.

"Vera?"

"Yes, Jim."

"What's your story?"

Kurt's hands tightened on the wheel and the Impala slid into the tunnel darkness, millions of gallons of water above us, heaving down in a long curve, like a bow with the string pulled, and above that, out of sight, the sky and the birds.

five

I sit on the bed, dressed. It is morning. The woman in white is busy around me, doing what I don't know, but the shade is open and I can see out the window into the street. Two boys, their backpacks riding low, walk toward school, I suppose. I have a recollection of such scenes. The boys disappear around a corner and the street is quiet for a moment until a car comes and a woman steps out her front door and onto the sidewalk. She seems late for something, running unsteadily in high heels, her body swaying.

"James, Eva is coming soon. She's taking you out. You'd better comb your hair."

The woman in white leads me away from the window and into the bathroom. The mirror shows my face. I look skeptical. I wet my hands and run them through my black-and-gray hair and then pull a comb through it. The woman in white says I look handsome, but I feel wet and lost and I want to know about the face in the mirror, my face, the one that is still there, but somehow hiding in bones and skin that ever so slightly have changed through the years to look a little like Kurt but mostly, I suppose, like me when I was younger. But I am not young and this is the face I've become, settled into. I feel like a dream in stone. The lady in white brushes my shoulder and slides a pen into my shirt pocket.

"You're a writer, James. A journalist. You wrote about things all over the world."

"What things?"

She holds newspaper stories with my name on the top. She says that's me. James Ryan.

"Mmmmm," I say.

I sense this explanation happens every day. It seems repeated but I can't be sure. The woman in white recites it like an actor saying her lines, or a person talking to a fool, bright and cheery, rehearsed, a mantra perhaps.

"Tell me about Kurt and Vera, James."

"What about them?"

"Everything. You took a trip with them. A long trip to the shore."

"An adventure, Kurt called it. Virginia Beach."

The woman in white sits on the bed with a folded shirt in her arms.

"And Vera. What was she like?"

"Enchanting. That's how Kurt described her to me once. We were sitting on our back stoop the second night after we met Vera and that's what he said. I agreed with him. It was funny, though, because Kurt never used that kind of word before. I knew all kinds of words back then. I looked them up in a dictionary my mother gave me one Christmas. Kurt thought it was an odd gift to give a kid."

"Tell me more about Vera. Was she pretty?"

"She could change on you like light through stained glass. Her hair was long and dark and her cheeks were high, her eyes restless. Her hands fluttered around her words and her fingers were long, almost translucent, and she wore spoon and amber rings that rattled on tabletops and car doors. She was great at thumb wrestling. I wanted to kiss her once. Not in a romantic way. She was in the kitchen. It was almost dark. She was squeezing grapefruits into a pitcher and she seemed scared or lost and I thought if I kissed her on the forehead she'd be okay. But I didn't. I just watched her for a while. When you were with Vera it seemed all the other sounds in the world went quiet. Did you ever know someone like that?"

The woman in white walks with a folded shirt to the window. Her back is to me; I think she says something, but I cannot be sure. There's a knock. The door opens and a lady steps in.

"Hi, Eva," says the woman in white, turning from the window.

The lady called Eva kisses me on the cheek and then on the forehead.

"He had a good night."

I am being talked about in the third person. I may be an idiot, but this much I know.

"James, I am Eva, your wife. I'm taking you on a ride to the beach. You love the beach."

"It's cold."

"You like it best in the cold. The cold and the gray, you used to say."

They hand me a coat. The woman holds my hand. Her hand is warm and firm; it slides nicely into mine. We step into the hallway, and the woman in white, from behind us, yells "good-bye," and we walk and I smell disinfectant. The scent passes and the front door opens and Eva, that is her name, and I descend the stone stairs and into the gray light, which she says I like and find inspiration from, which she says she always found strange, a man being moved and inspired by a sky the color of granite.

"That's from spending so much time in Eastern Europe, James. I think there's cloud and drizzle in your bones."

"The Berlin Wall."

"Yes, James. The Wall. See, sometimes you do come back, you do remember. I know you can remember more. You'll come back. You're just a little confused now, but you'll come back."

The lady kisses me on the lips. I feel like a dog that has learned a new trick. But I can tell in the lady's eyes that she means it; I am lost and she has come to bring me back, from where and to where I don't know, and she kisses me again, hard, and I have to say, I do like the way she tastes and feels and I seem to know her the way you know a character in an old storybook. The lady opens the door to a red Fiat Spider convertible.

"Remember? It's yours. But it's falling apart. Too many miles and rust around the back wheels. Look, the top is worn right here. "

I drop into the seat and close the door. Other scents. Cigarettes, mint, the perfume the lady is wearing, dampness and lemon, maybe from wood polish. Eva, she tells me her name is Eva, starts the car and we're off. I like sitting low like this, close to the ground, the tug of speed and gravity. Eva turns a corner and the back of the Fiat shimmies on the wet street, and she looks at me and rolls her eyes, and I think this must have happened a million times, but I can't be sure and so I look out the window at the stubby stoops and squat row houses and out to the wide boulevard and along a river and toward factory smoke and a bridge, which the lady tells me leads to the Jersey Shore. I know this. I know this geography.

I know Bob Dylan's on the tape player, but I don't know exactly what I'm doing here or why this lady in the driver's seat, who has just shifted into fifth gear, wants part of me, is driving me somewhere. I feel like a guy who showed up on the wrong night at the wrong theater trying to make sense of the scenery and strange faces coming out of the wings. Bob Dylan sings about leopard-skin pants and pill-box hats, and his is a voice you won't forget, no matter how much of your own life you've forgotten. It's a voice whistling through bone, rattling and whining as if it's fighting its own sound, daring beauty to be a mongrel. Very unlike the voice of Walter Jackson. My feet are cold. We're on the Atlantic City Expressway. The lady pulls off at a rest stop.

"I need a cigarette, James. Can't take Europe out of the girl."

She blows smoke through the crack in the window, a bit of drizzle on her face. I like this sky, this grayness. It mutes.

"It was like this all across Eastern Europe that year. Cold, dim, governments falling around us. Remember how we had to search every night to find an open phone line, one with no static, so you could send your stories back to the paper? You were an expert with alligator clips, taking apart the phone jacks in our hotel rooms, twisting wires to get your connection. Remember that? Sometimes you'd curse through the night because you couldn't get a connection to get your story out."

She crushes her cigarette in the ashtray, rolls the window down, and throws it out, a flash of lipstick brightening the gray. I seem to have this memory from someplace else, but it's gone and the lady waves smoke from the car and checks the mirror. She is graceful. I would not say elegant, but graceful. She pulls her dark hair back and ties it. Her face is a small sea of white, made fainter by lipstick and blue eyes; the blue of the earth seen from the moon. They come at you, inquisitive, not threatening. She says she is my lover, my wife; the one who raced through history with me and laughed with me amid the coal-stained hotels and icy bedrooms of Eastern Europe. She says the curtains in those rooms were brocaded, thick as blankets, letting in no light, even at midday. It was Charles Dickens, only gloomier, but somehow, at that time, along the lines of that changing map, it was the best place to be. If this happened, as she says it did, wouldn't I know? Some shred, some bright rag of memory? How can I not reach back to something so immediate in her voice? Am I that scoured of who I was?

"They brought him into the streets of Bucharest, James. Remember that? His scared ashen face, the face that had terrified so many. There it was among the bare trees and rifles of winter. In his coat, looking more like a doorman than a dictator. They tried him and then shot him on the cobblestones. You typed all night on that story. That image. You wanted to get it so right."

She leans over and kisses me. She starts the car and we are on the highway, past pines and sandy fringes, through a tollbooth and into traffic that thins as we head toward skeletal splays of neon hanging unlit from buildings in the mist. We come to the final stoplight, the beach and the pier ahead of us, gray compressing the horizon beyond the dark rocks of the jetty. The waves don't roll to the shore; they lunge, out of rhythm, breaking hard, white foam chasing spindly legged birds over the sand. This I do remember, this beach of childhood, of Kurt with his workingman's sunburn, his beer can half buried in the sand, his legs white with Coppertone, and Vera sitting in one of those low canvas chairs under an umbrella, reading the romantic parts of a book out loud to Kurt, who sometimes laughed but mostly shook his head. I see them out there. I want to go to them, me now in this old state, but I know when I get to where they're sitting, they'll be gone.

"Let's walk, James."

She takes my hand. We're careful on the slippery boardwalk. The shops are shuttered. I breathe in the dying-autumn scents of funnel cakes and taffy. She wraps her arms around mine, puts her head on my shoulder. There's a crack of sunlight in the gray. It shines on the sea, making a streak of blue through the green; the water is clean this time of year, unsettled but pure. A surfer bobs two hundred yards offshore. The water that far out is calm, the waves undefined, rolling, slowly finding form. The surfer waits. One wave then the next. Patient and cold, he spots that lift of water rising shadow-like behind him. He paddles. The wave catches him and they are one, and suddenly he's up, the board racing ahead of the wave, skimming through the curl, and the surfer disappears for a moment, but then his head breaks through the white and the wave crashes around him, an explosion of water, and he tumbles into the surf, his board twirling in the air like a broken airplane wing. He rises from the water, shiny in his wet suit, shivering and laughing. I feel I can hear him laughing in the wind.

"Sit here, James."

She lays plastic on the wet bench. She pulls a bottle of wine from her bag, two glasses and a corkscrew.

"Vranac. You must remember Vranac. From Montenegro. Good,

cheap wine; we drank it all across the Balkans. There's a shop in New York that sells it. I saw it in their window the other day. The same label. It's more expensive now. I guess the Balkans have become exotic. Mass graves and grapevines. Those graves, James, I still think about them. Rotting belts and tangled bones, you wrote. I think we used to pay five Deutsche Marks a bottle back then. Here."

I sip.

"Maybe your taste will remember what your mind cannot."

I sip again, but no. It is good, but it brings nothing back, awakens no ghosts.

She lifts a fat envelope from her bag and thumbs through it.

"These are some of my favorite stories of yours, James. I keep them with me wherever I go. They're getting brittle and yellow. I should laminate them, but I like the feel of the paper. Let's see. Here's a good one. MERCHANT OF DEATH KILLED AT SEA."

His name was Goran, a Croatian fisherman who moonlighted as a gunrunner and a spy. He was basketball-big the way Croats are, a swoop of black hair hanging over his brow. He knew all the islands off the coast, and at night Eva and I would meet him and go trawling through the darkness, him cutting his engines while through infrared binoculars we saw guns and grenades loaded onto boats that slipped back to shore to waiting trucks that drove through Split and Mostar on their way to Sarajevo. We drank plum brandy on the boat and watched how the world worked, foreign voices, the slosh of the sea, the bang and clatter of crates, money passed, new meeting times set, the throaty sounds of engines accelerating away from the islands, silhouettes in the starlight. Goran had a daughter. She sunbathed topless when he fished. She was twenty, a student before the war. Her father sent her near the Serb lines to seduce. She was good at it, and she helped Goran put dots and lines on maps.

They lived in a whitewashed and shuttered house on the cliffs above the sea. The house had been in the family for hundreds of years, and Goran said from the window you could feel like God, watching the tides tug and pull at the shore. Goran said the window view was best in winter when snow squalls blew over the sea and whirled up the cliffs, spinning around his house and up to heaven. I supposedly asked Goran about heaven, and he laughed, saying only Croats were admitted. It is the great trick of Croats on humanity, he said. The world thinks everyone has a chance at heaven, that heaven is a place filled with souls from every country, but this is not so; heaven flies only the Croat flag, and is very small.

We slept at Goran's house and the next day, hours after we had left, Eva and I stopped at a gas station and found that Goran had slipped a case of Vranac into the trunk. There was a note. "Before the war, this was my favorite wine. But it is made by Serbs and I have no taste for it now."

Eva and I traveled to Sarajevo and stayed a month. We decided to take a break from the fighting after a mortar round burst through our window but didn't explode. When we went back over the mountains to Croatia, villagers reported that Goran and his daughter had been killed. His boat went adrift one night, struck the rocks off an island, and sank. Their bodies were found the next morning, throats slit, bullet wounds to temples, floating in a cove. They were buried in the rocky earth near Goran's house. The story in my hands was written in the first person, supposedly by me. Did I really know a gunrunner and his spy daughter? Did I scribble their lives in a notebook? I hand the story back to the lady. She folds it into a fat envelope.

"I came to this beach once with Kurt and Vera. Then we went to another beach in Virginia. That's the beach I know most, what happened there. It was long ago. Did you know about Kurt and Vera?"

"Yes, James. I know all about them."

"They're clearest in my mind. The rest is not there. I see this bottle. I read Vranac, but it may as well be a rocket ship. I know I've lost something; every now and then an image goes through my head, something that I've seen, but before I can place it, it's gone."

"Place me, James. Feel my face in your hand. Something in you must know, a tissue, a nerve. How can all those days, months, years vanish from you? I keep asking the doctors, how? Wonderful explanations they give. Did they tell you the one about your mind as a glacier, with fissures and light and some such drivel. They don't know. Medicine doesn't know, James."

I sip wine. It's warm and it's not such a pain sitting in the wet with this lady.

"Eva. Say my name, James. Eva."

"Eva."

"I'm going to ask you later what my name is and you're going to say Eva."

"Okay."

A surfer battles against the shore waves and paddles through to calmer water. Deep and cold, a swirl beneath him, the unseen power of the earth, a mystery of conspiring elements. Creation in a ball, flung into orbit. The wine is good. The lady pours me another glass. The rain falls hard but we don't move. She holds my hand. The surfer sits in the sea, the point of his board bobbing like a flash of fin. The lady whispers to me about another time she wants me to remember, and it all sounds wonderful, exciting. I like the rain on my face. It's cold and I have a chill. I don't want to move. I want to sit here and finish this bottle of wine, and what's wrong with that? This is what I know now. I see the glass. I see the wine. I taste. This is who I am. Now.

"The communists were scattered and scared. They knew . . ."

The surfer finds his wave.

"We thought there'd be tanks, like before, like in '68 . . ."

He's up.

"Hardly a shot was fired. We went from city to city. Champagne and barbed wire . . ."

The wave lifts quickly, steep, sharp.

"They were waiting for magic . . ."

The surfer slices down the folding water.

"Democracy and capitalism will save us . . ."

Faster he moves.

"A new vocabulary spread overnight across half a continent . . ."

He's in the curl.

"A wall fell. New faces with new power. The unimaginable before us . . ."

He's lost.

"You wrote about it, James. Every day for months . . ."

He's free of the curl, racing along the wave's last remnant.

"An era ended. The missiles in their silos. It can happen, the impossible."

The surfer rides to shore, standing, he doesn't fall.

"What a time, James . . ."

He picks up his board and jogs toward a twisted towel in the sand.

"C'mon. We're soaked. We have a hotel room down the beach."

He takes the towel and walks, shrinking in the distance.

"Okay, James. What's my name?"

I cannot answer her.

Eva's going to keep him out tonight. She does that sometimes, tries to spill herself into him, compressing all their years into hours. Maybe it'll bring him back. Maybe the mention of Prague or Budapest at the right time in the pitch of night will glow across his synapses and become as real to him as Kurt and Vera. I pray for his tangled brain to see. It can happen. There are miracles. A miracle led me to James. He and I are forever entwined.

Before she died, and what a sad way it was, Vera told me in a letter barbed with notations and thick as a book that she was my mother and Kurt my father. It was a startling revelation; a voice echoing across time. The letter was kept from me for many years. It lay in a taped box beneath a floorboard hidden by a Persian carpet in a small house in New England. I had walked over that carpet all my life and never knew that just below my feet was the story of how I came to be. Secrets, though, like air bubbles, wriggle their way to the surface. When I finally read it, Vera had been dead a long while, but her words, ahhh her words, coiled through me and found home. "This tale, my daughter, is for you." Is there a sweeter phrase? Page after page, Vera whispered to me. I pieced her story together and made a map of words and memories that led me to James. My half-brother doesn't know this side of Kurt and Vera. Things changed, were altered back when he was a boy, and by the time he became a man, and his name went from Jim to James, he had no inkling. Why would he? We were orphans in different places, children of worlds that touched briefly and bounced away. The letter told me this. Yet there is still much I do not know. Imagine you have a life but then you discover you have another that lies in the murk of an addled man's mind. My story lives inside his darkness. James must remember more. I wait. I perch like a blackbird on a branch, patient for lost trinkets and flashes of tin.

When James is out like this with Eva, I come to his room and sit in the moonlight. The halls are quiet, the deranged sedated and tucked away for the night — it's amazing how the muddled brain can slumber — and the only sound is the occasional shuffle of nurse shoes on polished floors or pills spilled across a counter, drumming like rain on a roof.

I read James's newspaper stories and try to put myself in those moments of history. It will bring us closer if I can experience them the way he did: NO SHOTS FIRED IN CZECH "VELVET REVOLUTION." SLEDGEHAMMERS, FREEDOM BREAK OPEN BERLIN WALL. ROMANIAN PRESIDENT EXECUTED BY FIRING SQUAD. And my favorite, from a village in the Balkans, A BOY'S JOURNEY THROUGH WAR TO MANHOOD AND, FINALLY, DEATH. I try to imagine beyond the words, like when you read a book and you sense another world happening that doesn't exist on the page but exists because of the page, and that makes it true and part of the story.

James's story is my secret. I almost told it to the owner of the corner market, Earl, who watches me in the aisles and knows I prefer paper to plastic. He has a nasal voice and a lazy eye but he alerts me to specials on pastrami, pickles, toilet paper, and milk. The big chains, says Earl, are killing the small grocer; he may sell out one day to a dry cleaner or a tattoo parlor. Earl's had offers. We chat about family. Earl's quite open about such things; he's the kind of misbegotten soul they invite on afternoon talk shows, earnest and giving of details most would prefer to keep private: Vietnam flashbacks, estranged wives, a son's suicide, a stint in jail, a recidivist 12-Stepper. He mixes highs and lows like a brawler in a Tom Waits song and sometimes I imagine him sitting in a small apartment and weeping through the night until dawn. But there is something about Earl. With his white smock and pocket of pens, his slow rhythm of ringing up prices on an ancient cash register, Earl has a tenderness I find rare in this world.

"What's your brother do?" he asked the other day.

"He was a famous journalist. He's retired now."

"You see him much?"

"Every day."

"I wish I was that close to my sister."

I left it at that. It was a pretty thought.

I go to James's window and point my face toward the moon, feeling its crystal, cool light and studying my reflection in the glass: a mirage dressed in white, the circle of my stethoscope shining, my face as faint as fog, my hair pulled back, my deep-set eyes, James's eyes, shadowed like caves at the forest's edge. I seem a girl at a dance, a picture in a locket, an image, frozen. I run my fingers over my name tag, tracing the letters and looking out over the city, James's boyhood city, the city my mother, the "enchanting" Vera, escaped to on a summer night of rainstorms and lightning.

seven

"Vera, what's your story?"

I yelled into the dark wind of the Chesapeake Bay Bridge Tunnel. Kurt accelerated and the bay pressed down in its arc over us. We raced toward the square of light at the tunnel's end, the Impala roaring back into the day. I squinted in the sun; a spit of beach in the distance, the gray hulks of navy ships sailing heavy and low toward Norfolk. Vera stood up in the car like a lady general, holding on to the windshield, her black hair blowing as if painted against the sky. She screamed something into the wind, but I couldn't hear what it was. She sat down and held my hand. Kurt reached for the radio, but Vera slapped him away and laughed and said let the day and the wind and the bay and the birds speak for themselves. Kurt shook his head and I sat between them on the front seat as we came off the bridge and the Impala, gas dropping toward E and temperature leaning toward H, rolled onto the sandy plains of Virginia.

"My story is a long one, Jim."

That was all she said. She opened her purse and pulled the rearview mirror toward her, shading on lipstick and eyeliner, smoothing her hair, and disappearing behind her sunglasses like someone incognito. We drove a stretch of highway and came to a road of traffic lights leading toward Virginia Beach. You could smell summer: cotton candy, popcorn, french fries, snow cones, tanning oil, all mingling, metastasizing (a good dictionary word) around us like we were in another place, a new planet. The Jersey Shore near Philly was similar in summer, but it was more exotic in the South; it seemed summer was more at home here, more relaxed and welcoming. Kurt pulled into a 7-Eleven and bought us Slurpees, cola for me, cherry for Vera, and a lime for him. I listened to the people going in and out of the store; they held on to syllables longer, their consonants were softer, their words seemed to float, especially the words of three girls who walked into the 7-Eleven in their bikinis, sand on their brown shoulders, their long hair damp and flat against their backs. Kurt saw me watching.

"Hey, Jim, why don't we ask those girls if they want to play miniature golf? There's all kinds of miniature golf down here. Volcanoes, gorillas."

I blushed and sucked on my Slurpee.

"We can wait for those girls to come out, Jim. They're probably getting Slurpaaaays, too."

"Listen to Kurt with his new accent," said Vera. "Take me to your plantation, sir."

"Let's just go," I said.

Kurt and Vera laughed. As we backed up, the girls stood at the counter, their brown fingers sliding coins to a clerk in a red shirt. Kurt turned on the radio again. The Jackson Five. When Michael sang about something as lowly as a rat, it calmed you, made you think of something religious. I closed my eyes, the sun warm on my face and arms, my hair windblown and feeling like straw, the Impala moving slow in the traffic. Kurt's patience could be measured in centimeters, but this traffic, which would normally have him squirming and cursing, didn't bother him; he sat there sweating and humming to songs as Vera uncapped silver nail polish and, leaning over me, painted a star, the kind you got for getting an A on an arithmetic exam, on his cheek. Kurt found a parking spot after he bargained with a guy. We pulled the top to the Impala shut and Vera chased me out of the car. She hung a towel in the window and changed into her bathing suit. I thought it would be a bikini, but it wasn't, it was a sky-blue one-piece that made her legs longer. She put on an old fedora and one of

Kurt's buttondown shirts bought years earlier when he thought he might look for a job with a desk and an air conditioner. He never found one, but I don't think he searched too hard. I had to admit, I never could have imagined him coming home from work without scratches on his arms and ship rust in his hair. We followed Vera over a small dune through tall, itchy grass to where the sand tapered to the beach. The waves were green and white-tipped, kites snapped in the air, and Vera threw down a blanket near the edge of where the last wave rolled up the farthest.

"It's cooler down here."

"Tide's changing. We'll have to keep moving the blanket."

"I don't mind."

I hadn't noticed before, but Vera had a scar on the side of her upper right thigh. Hard and white, it was the size of a quarter, round and a little ragged, like Pluto through a telescope. Vera held a transistor radio to her ear and Kurt slept facedown on the blanket. She rubbed lotion on his back with her free hand and burrowed her feet into the sand. I walked toward the pier. It was crooked, pilings were missing, and the wood was ancient and dark. It was like a shipwreck without sails; a splintered galleon from a history book. Surfers shot through the pilings, shadowed for a moment, and then zipped with the wave into the sun. Their girlfriends sat on the beach, laughing and squeezing lemons over their hair; maybe it was the southern sun, but the girls here tanned better than the ones up north, the color was even, natural, a second tempting skin. One of them waved to me but I kept moving. The air beneath the pier cooled and I walked on. The dunes slumped closer to the beach, blankets were fewer, and I imagined an unchartered country, a stretch touched only by God. Like at the end of *Planet of the Apes* when Charlton Heston comes upon the Statute of Liberty toppled on the shore; both he and the statue, looking sideways at him from the sand, seem confused, and Heston realizes that the alien planet his spaceship landed on was really earth in the way, way distant future, like starlight shooting backward, and all he ever knew and loved before was gone. Buckets, kids, a woman with a white robe and glass of iced tea waved to a man who stood in the blurry heat of a charcoal fire on the porch of a big house. I looked to the horizon. Vera's world was out there, the silk bazaars and desert fires and farther east the Nile Delta, where Moses, according to the Bible and Fr. Heaney, was set adrift in a basket. I glanced back toward the pier and saw Vera walking toward me, passing through the shadows, her bathing suit flashing like blue magic.

"What's your story, Jim?"

"It's a small one."

"I left Kurt sleeping. When the wave hits the blanket he'll wake up quick."

Vera laughed, playing it out in her head. She stood beside me. I felt Kurt's shirt brush my arm. The surf swirled around our ankles. Pelicans raced in dark succession over the ocean, their wing tips inches from the waves; farther out fishing boats waddled silently where the water met the sky, reminding me of tin ducks at a carnival shooting stand. The bay we had crossed earlier was salty, tangy, tamed, almost restful with its bulrush and bone-gray trees, but this ocean was wild and pure and rough, its colors changing with sun and cloud from blue to deep blue to green to the foaming white edge of the wave's curl. The waves struck the beach and pulled back, rushing out to their deep, hidden source, moving in warm and cool currents, invisible serpents. I ran from Vera and jumped into a wave, my body slicing through the water, feeling the pressure and the tug, the immense weight, and then surfacing, water running off me, shining in the sun, my face warm until another wave knocked and rolled me, my back scraping the sand, stinging and cool, and laughing with my mouth closed beneath the water, surrendering to its power. I walked out, dripping, toward Vera. I shook my wet hair.

She squealed and pushed me away. We stood looking at each other, smiling; me young and sand-scraped in the light, and Vera, her back to the dunes, her face toward the ocean. What is that word when all seems right, when a moment marks itself in you somewhere and you keep it? Resplendent. My dictionary called it resplendent.

"Let's swim to the other side."

"You've been there."

"I'll go back. You go, too, Jim. See what's out there. So much. There was a church in Carthage on the cliffs. It had clinging vines and loose stones. The mosaics were fading. In the afternoons an old man would walk up the hill and play piano in the church. I never knew what he was playing, but the notes rolled out of that old church and over the sea and for all I knew they kept going and never quieted. I sat there many afternoons listening to that old man's music and watching far-off boats. Can you picture it?"

"Yeah. It's like in the near sunset, when a guy's on his stoop, drinking a beer and smoking a cigar and listening to the Phillies on the radio. You can smell the aftershave coming off him and hear his wife inside through the screen door. It's as if his day is done and for a couple of hours he lives inside that radio."

"Those are the things you carry forever, Jim. Those scents and sounds."

Vera walked back from the water and sat in the sand. I sat with her. Late-afternoon clouds, white, not threatening, hung before us. Sand crabs skittered; the tide crept up. Vera rubbed her scar.

"Sometimes it itches. It's hard like a stone. Feel it."

She was right.

"It's part of my story, Jim."

"You don't have to tell me."

"I thought you wanted to know."

"I do, but a scar like that, I guess, is personal. I just don't know why we're on this trip or where we're going."

The man was from Marrakesh. He was not a spice merchant; he was a rich man's son Vera had met in a tea shop. He said he was a jeweler, but he was a smuggler, a man who traded diamonds and guns across Africa. He was tall and lean with long muscles and he moved, Vera said, as if he never touched the ground. He fed her pomegranates and saffron rice. Vera had been traveling with friends, but she stayed behind in Marrakesh with the man until she found out all of his lies, or most of them, or enough to spoil what was once enticing. She left one night and he came looking. He found her in Casablanca.

She ran away again and he tracked her down in Rabat, where he shot her with a small pistol on a drunken night; a woman doctor dug out the bullet, cleaned the wound, and stitched her. Vera said she remembered the way the brownish antiseptic mixed with the blood, turning her skin yellow and sepia like a strange vegetable under the steel examining room light. The doctor told her to escape and said Vera didn't understand that she had become a trapped prize; a woman with fair skin and blue eyes on the North African coast was precious. Like a diamond to be possessed but never loved.

Vera made her way to Spain and flew home to the Cleveland suburb where her father sold Cadillacs and winter came in hard and the scenery was so changed from Marrakesh that she felt safe, as if delivered to a new shore with no trace of that other world. But the man began appearing, in a mirror, a store window, a distant figure on a sidewalk. She felt him everywhere: the shadow behind her in the movie theater, the stranger with his face hidden by a newspaper in a café. The man, his name was Mounir, hovered but never arrived, as if he wanted to haunt, like a wild dog slinking through tall grass on the African plains before it strikes. Vera said he would kill her; she was sure of it. She ran again.

She had been running seven months, the bullet wound, once spreading like a purple bloom beneath her skin, healed to a raised white scar. That's when she met Kurt and me in the Philly diner and came home with us that night. She said the man had been tracking her across alleys and that she hid in a church, scrunched down behind the altar, and then slipped out through the vestibule to the street where she spotted Kurt and me in the window. Maybe, she said, it was the light over the table, but from the outside Kurt and I seemed like people she could trust, and when she came in and sat with us, she looked at Kurt's hands, hard and battered from sand-blasting and painting ships, and knew he would offer sanctuary. She said they were strong hands, solid and coarse enough to keep even a gun smuggler from Marrakesh away. That's what she thought; that's all she wanted, a pair of steady hands to keep her safe.

She had not seen the man since she'd been with us, although driving down the Eastern Shore, she thought she glimpsed him behind us in an El Dorado that turned and vanished in the road dust. Vera stopped her story. She put her chin on her knees and looked at the ocean. She leaned on me and we sat in the sand. The waves were cold and clean, hitting the shore hard, mist rising, the way it does just before night when the tide and the air change and new creatures scatter over the sand.

I didn't know what to think of Vera's story. It was more mysterious than even the best Lizabeth Scott movie, and I bet Kurt, if he knew the tale, which he must, felt he was in a script, on the lam, and protecting a girl with a bullet in her past. I supposed that would intrigue Kurt, that late-night, movie-watching side of him, anyway. The mark was there on Vera's leg. It looked like a bullet scar would look, and Vera did know about spices and desert windstorms and Marrakesh with its colors, balconies, and flowers mixing in with boats and nets and fishermen hunched over hash wisps from shisha pipes. But why does a man like the one she described spend all his time following her and doing nothing? I looked behind me and down the beach. Was a stranger with an accent and a small pistol roaming the coming night? I squinted but saw nothing. Then a figure moved under the pier and headed toward us: Kurt, cursing, sandy, his blanket drenched.

"I was sleeping and the wave hit me and washed my beer away."

Vera laughed. I laughed, too. Kurt's cutoffs hung damp and heavy at his waist. He grabbed Vera, threw her on his shoulders, and twirled her toward the waves. She screamed and laughed and told Kurt he had better put her down, but he kept twirling, getting dizzy, losing his knees, wobbling as the water rushed up on him and then he tumbled into a big wave with Vera, and for a moment they were gone, and then Vera popped up and then Kurt. She walked over and pushed him back into the water and another wave came and knocked them both into the shore and they popped up again, beaten and tired and Vera grabbed Kurt and held him and jumped up in his arms and he carried her out of the waves, and she seemed small, thin, her black hair matted in strands, as if the waves had washed some of her away. We walked under the pier and toward our car. Kurt carried Vera the entire way. She tried to teach us a few words of Arabic, the throaty, clipped syllables made the night exotic. Inshallah — God willing. Allahu Akbar — God is great. Hasbyallah wa ne'malwakil — I complain to God, He is my best resort. God is in the language, Vera said; he lives in Arabic more than he does in English.

"A different God," said Kurt.

"Same God, different name," said Vera. "He's a desert god, ruler of a harsh place."

Kurt opened the Impala's trunk and tossed us towels. We drove to a hotel and the girl at the counter — she looked no older than me — said, "Do y'all need a room?" Y'all was so much softer than Vera's Arabic; it was a word that didn't come at you so much as rolled over and through you. The girl pinged a silver bell on the counter and a little, bent man appeared and grabbed our two suitcases. He walked toward the elevator, his right foot splayed as if unhinged, and the girl whispered to us, "He's my uncle. He ain't right in the head if you know what I mean. But Daddy's gotta take care of him. Kin is kin, after all. But he's good for carrying things and he'll show you to your rooms."

The elevator opened on the fifth floor and you could faintly hear the Beach Boys, tinny, every note false, from the transistor in the lobby. Kurt and Vera took 501 and the bent man led me to 503. Vera came in and gave the man two quarters and he handed me the key and disappeared. Vera kissed me on the cheek and ran off to 501. My room's balcony overlooked the ocean. It was night. The sand was gray from up here and the ocean black. Lights glowed on the faraway horizon, floating in the air, unattached, like spirits, but I knew they were the lights of freighters and trawlers that sailed beyond. A man leaned over the boardwalk railing nearest the hotel. He looked out to sea and then turned and looked at the hotel, up its floors as if he were staring right at me, and then looked away again to the sea. I went inside and closed the curtains.

The phone rang. "How y'all doing? Rooms okay? Can I gitcha anything?" I said thank you and no. I took a shower, the warm water tasted like salt. I dressed and watched TV. A knock on the door.

"Hey, I came to check on you. Need towels. Soap?" said the girl from the desk.

"No. Well, maybe an extra towel if you have any."

She laughed. "You wanna make out? I'm a good kisser. But only kissing. Some of you boys want more but I only kiss."

She was blond and wore white shorts and a forest-green halter top. She stepped in and wrapped her arms around me and started kissing me; her lips were shiny and smelled of cinnamon. She pressed hard and her teeth clinked my teeth but then she eased and kissed some more and it was strange and nice, and I don't know why, but I closed my eyes and kissed her back and we fell on the bed and she landed on top of me. She had a short, hard tongue, and she was light

54

upon me. She sat up and straightened her hair. "I better git down to the desk. My uncle's down there; he gets confused after a while. Maybe I'll come back later and we'll kiss some more. But only kissing. Some guy from Massachusetts the other week wanted more and I said, 'No sir, buddy.' I'm a Baptist and I don't need that on my soul. Kissing's okay, though. Mr. Jones, our Bible group leader, says kissing teaches, what's that word, uh, moderation, that's it, moderation and maturity. If you're here next week — I can't tell how long you'll be here because your daddy, he is your daddy, right? 'Cuz one time we had a kidnapped boy here with a terrible man. The police came. — Anyway, there's this special preacher coming all the way up from Charlotte to give a sermon on young people and love. My daddy says he's a mighty fine preacher. Are you a Baptist? You're not a Jew, are you? My daddy says stay away from Jews. I better git."

She left.

That was the second time I made out with a girl. It was nice to have it happen unexpected. My first make-out was with Carmen Pasquele at night in an alley beyond a summer stickball game. I was batting fifth and Carmen, whom I had held hands with two days earlier, came along and whispered for me to follow her. I knew what was coming and I got a little knotted as I walked past Stan's Deli and the truck repair shop and into the alley, where Carmen leaned back on the wall and pulled me to her and kissed me so soft that I barely felt it, but I did and it went right through me like a sip of hot chocolate slipping down your throat and spreading through your chest. She kissed me again and I heard the thwack of our fourth batter, Billy Holmes, and Carmen knew and she said, "Go back to your game, Jim." She kissed me on the cheek and went the other way down the alley, her sandals scraping the road and her dress so short you had to wonder what Carmen was actually hiding up there.

The phone rang. I thought it might be the girl from the front desk, but it was Kurt.

"We eat in five minutes."

I shut off the light and went out on the balcony. The man on the boardwalk was gone and the thrum of the waves hypnotized me, washing in a thought and carrying it away, then washing in another one. I looked over and saw Vera sitting on the balcony of 501. She was in the dark, too, her cigarette ember moving like a lazy firefly. She wore a white dress that made her incandescent against the night and the moon, like those jellyfish that glow in the cold, cold deep of the ocean. She was crying, her body a ripple of slow shakes, swallowing her sound so Kurt wouldn't hear.

She didn't see me on the balcony of 503. I blended in with the night. The break of the waves hid my breathing. Kurt came up behind her. He kissed her neck and rubbed her shoulders. Vera turned into him, and it seemed like a scene from our kitchen back in Philly years ago when Kurt held my mom in the darkness after dinner, when they thought I was asleep, but I was awake on the stairs watching their shadows dance on the wall from headlights passing in the alley. Kurt held Vera like a lover, but also like he was holding himself and, to me, he was newborn in the darkness.

The trip had already changed him. The scent of paint and turpentine no longer trailed him, the bay and the ocean healed the cuts and nicks on his hands; fresh skin grew over the scrapes on his forearms. He walked less like a workingman and more like a man indifferent to the world. The order he had once known, which had kept the bills in his wallet layered in sequential order and the Impala buffed and shined, no longer mattered, or at least seemed less immediate, less pervasive. He was half shaven and uncombed, this new creature, my father. His tennis clothes were rumpled, but his game stayed sharp, and if you wanted to see the old Kurt you sat near the baseline and watched the squeak and slide of his feet, the butterfly stroke of his backhand. He kept his tenderness, the way he dipped his head and whispered a word when he wanted you to glimpse what was in his heart; Vera drew that out in him the way a hot pin gives rise to a splinter wedged deep.

He had been tender with Mom, but Mom didn't need a protector, except on that day the Fleetwood slid on ice, skipped the sidewalk, and flew toward her. I was in school. Kurt was at work, breaking frost off a freighter. Mom died in a snow pile, surrounded by the faces of neighbors and strangers that hung like lanterns in the late-morning winter light. I went with him to O'Malley's Funeral Home the night they delivered Mom from the morgue. We sat in two big chairs, both of us stone-still, every creak and sound in that old house striking through us. O'Malley called us in to see Mom. A white sheet pulled to her chin, lilies in a clear vase on a table. I waited, and I think Kurt did, too, for her to wake so we could carry her home and she could finish the cake she was baking, but she didn't stir, and O'Malley rubbed his small, speckled hand over Kurt's back and Kurt put his arm around me and I felt the snow in my boot treads melt into the gold carpet. Kurt bent over and kissed Mom. I kissed her, too, on the forehead, and as I pulled back my eyes caught the tunnel of a lily, white and winter-cold, tiny crisscrosses of veins alive with water from O'Malley's tap.

We walked home. Snow fell, yet the sky was clear, and the moon was a fuzzy light and the footprints of the day were gone and streets and alleys lay before us like uncharted territory. Kurt reached down and held my hand. It was warm and wide as a mitten. We walked to the church and stood outside beneath the stained glass, peering through snowfall to amber, red, blue, burgundy, and the palest white, the bone-white of Christ un-nailed from the cross, His body draped like linen, His wounds, dried red slits, marking hands and feet and the place where the lance drew water and blood from His side. Kurt said he was confused. He said being a father and a husband were a singular thing to him, and he didn't know if he could be one without the other, but he would try. He wanted to stay out in the snow

57

all night. He didn't want to return to the house because it would be like coming home from a late shift and Mom's apron would be on the table and the scent of her would be there and there'd be a plate of something in the oven and the TV would be murmuring, or maybe she'd be in the bath or maybe out of the bath and reading in the backroom, her feet in those thick gray hunting socks she wore, or maybe she'd have fallen asleep and he'd have to tiptoe and stay quiet like a ghost, like he did on so many nights when she fell asleep, and he'd slip under the blanket feeling the trapped warmth of her burn through him like whiskey. Kurt didn't want to go home and not find that.

We left the church and walked past Veterans Stadium and all the way to the docks, where the ships floated like gray, rusted mountains on black water streaked with a few lights. Kurt told me about each ship, where it had been, the seas it had sailed, the repairs it needed, the clunk and steam of its engine and how he swung from ropes, painting its sides, his feet tap-dancing over the water. He spoke until dawn, never letting go of my hand. The sky that brought the moon was gone; the sun broke clear on the horizon, and the ships in the new day were less majestic than at night. We walked home.

Vera stopped crying and laughed into Kurt's chest. He pushed her hair back and wiped her eyes. They left the balcony. The muslin white curtain floated out of the sliding glass door and blew in the breeze. I didn't ask Kurt why he chose to sleep in Vera's room. I knew. Vera didn't remind Kurt of Mom or the house or our alley or his job; she was magic in the lamplight, with clothes and scents and stories from other places that allowed Kurt, and me, to leave behind, at least for a moment, the inklings of who we were. I stepped off my balcony and sat in the dark of the bed in Room 503, tasting cinnamon and bubble gum and waiting for Kurt's knock to go get something to eat.

eight

Eva Ryan.

She signs the ledger as Eva Ryan. The penmanship is clear, precise; the E and the R ornate as if they had been written by a breeze blowing through ink.

"Hello, Mr. Ryan."

I don't know this man behind the counter smiling at me, but like so much else, it seems as if I should, so I nod to him and smile back. My clothes are wet. I am cold. My shoes are sandy. The man hands the lady a key and a bellboy takes our small bags, leading us to a flight of stairs and down a half-lit corridor to a room that opens to the ocean, the sliding glass door filled with dimming light and white-limned waves in the distance. The bellboy leaves the bags and closes the door. The lady goes into the bathroom and I sit on the bed, wet, the taste of wine on my lips. It is dusk. The room is almost dark and the ocean slips away, a retreating lull spooling back to a faraway time zone. The woman comes out wrapped only in a towel and the bathroom light behind her makes her a silhouette, a shadow.

"Remember this room, James?"

I do not.

"We lived in this room for three months after Europe changed. You wrote your first book here. You hurried it. You made me read over your shoulder as you typed. The publisher wanted it quickly and this room was scattered with papers and pens and notes and room service trays and you wrote and wrote and the night you finished we ran to the beach with towels and a bottle of wine."

I do not. I do not. I do not. Remember.

"I am Eva, James."

She steps toward me, takes off her towel, and pats my face with it. She bends and slips off my shoes and peels off my clothes and dries me. Slowly. My skin is damp and cold, like the chill off a marble floor, and the woman and I slip under the covers, and the sheets are cool and she pulls me to her, my marble skin on her warmth and we are still, and I think I must know this; there is a shred of memory somewhere, perhaps in a capillary, or a vein buried deep. I have known this before. I feel it in me, but it is like a possession stolen, lost, left on a windowsill.

She takes my hand and then a finger and puts the finger on her forehead and moves it down her nose and over her lips and down her chin to her throat. I am tracing her, to her breasts and across her nipples. I feel her heartbeat and down I move; she's guiding me, over her belly and across her hips. She whispers that I must know this. I must know the shape of her, yes, she says, her body has changed with time, but still I must know, the bones and her spirit, the same, unchanged. She pulls the covers back. She lies in the last light of the day and what I have traced is a painting in a museum, the pale white of her body, a filament, a mirror before me; she wants me to see myself in the flesh and bone of her love. That's what she says. Love, in this bed, down a bellboy's corridor along the sea. She kisses me, and I know her, maybe not all of her, not every line of history she tells me we have, but of all the words she has spoken, and I guess there must have been many, it is this kiss that makes me see the forgotten places. I kiss her back.

"James?"

"Yes."

"Are you here?"

"I think."

"Hang on to it. Don't get lost again."

She kisses me and pulls me to her tight.

"Eva, where have I been?"

She doesn't answer. She squeezes me, presses me against her. What's real, her hair on the pillow, her lips on mine, is permanent, constant; as if I had gone to the bathroom in the night and returned to find things set right, her slumber, clothes draped over chairs, blankets and sheets riffled like the waves of the sea. This moment I know. Eva is Eva, but older. Perhaps I am writing a story, but where are we? All I know is this room and Eva. My notes, scribbled, disheveled, what do they say? I must go to the window, but Eva says no; the streets and alleys are quiet, there will be news tomorrow, but for now the news sleeps, the Havels and Walesas have returned to their vodkas and whispered asides. The revolution slumbers in damp coats and cigarette smoke; the pope is in the Vatican; Reagan and Gorbachev are toe-to-polished-toe; the world hangs on sound-bites and secret meetings. What comes tomorrow, we will see. I hear the roll of waves. Maybe, we are in Danzig, or as the Poles call it Gdansk, waiting for a protest amid blowtorch light and broken ships. Eva opens her arms. "You want to chase it, don't you? Chase what's out there in the dark and bring it back and put words to it." I don't feel like writing tonight. I fall into her and she laughs, Eva, older Eva, the imprint of her youth just below my fingers. Let me trace. Her face tighter, beauty stretched, and lines, just a few, as if drawn with a needle, float around mouth and eyes. The lips are full and the shoulders, oh the shoulders, the muscle beneath taut as the strings of a mandolin; all her power is there, imperceptibly bowed like a fighter stepping into his jab; the breasts and down to the hips, white as if rolled from flour, always so white she was, glowing in darkened rooms, and sometimes the black hair of her head and the black between her legs were one with the night as if a white figure was being pulled and formed from a sea of ink, and the wet warmth between those legs, that was Eva, and she is here, beneath me, in the trace and the touch, but when I move across her . . . suddenly, things shift and flash the way house lights flicker before a storm. I see Eva. I see a woman. I see Eva. I see . . . It goes. She sits up, pushes me back, turns on the nightstand light. She holds my face in her hands like a vase, her eyes looking through mine.

"You're slipping away. For a moment you were here. Do you remember?"

"The kiss. Something happened. But now I'm confused. Where are we?"

"The doctors say it comes like that. A moment of clarity. They call it 'triggers' and 'mechanisms' like the words for a machine. These clear moments will become fewer and then one day you won't find the path back, not by a kiss, not by a scent. Remembering has been briefer, James. When you come back now, you are like a man on a doorstep peeking into a house with your car running in the street. Where do you go when you run into the street? Why can't I follow and bring you back? Is it a fortress in there? I am Eva, James. Eva. We made love in rooms like this across the world, and now we are two bodies, separate. I feel like a beggar following you for change."

"Tell me more."

"I used to bring you back with a story. The time in Europe, a headline, one of your clippings, even a funny remembrance from a train or a border checkpoint, something that clicked inside you. They no longer evoke. I see your eyes; they have become the stories from a history book, not a life. You can't place yourself. It's as if the puzzle is done except for one piece, the piece you hold in your hand, but you can't see that the piece fits perfectly into the picture before you. Now it's only primal, James. I bring you back with this bed, our bodies. It's a straight line to the core, no words, no time to think or remember. Be still James, not confused. Touch me."

She takes my hand and moves it across her face and to her breasts and below. Warm, wet; the scent of her rising through the sheets, the scent on my fingertips to the nerve endings and into me, these elements to remember, and now I am on my back and she is over me and I am inside this warmth, this place I know, where all of Eva's nerves are alive; they pull me to her like a net and she is moving over me and her eyes she won't take off me; she is using her body in place of words, this strong body, older yes, but this body is what I know, it is my map and wherever I was, I am back now; the face before me is not a ghost from a scrapbook, not a gray clip from a newspaper, it is Eva, my rhythm, my light, and I know how much she loved sex, she craved it at day's end, even at day's middle, and it is this Eva over me now. She is crying and I am with her, there is no distance, no fog, no gauzy memory; this is the room I know, this hotel on the Jersey Shore, ninety minutes south of Philly, through the Pinelands and the sand grit, to the boys on the jetty, and Eva and I, here, in this room with the same key handed to us for years, and the empty bottle of Vranac on the table, and the mass graves of Bosnia and the fallen, rebuilt lands of Europe, all in this bed, brought back by Eva's will, her body, the warm, thick scent that covers me, and I reach up and feel her throat and her breath and she is at that moment when the eyes roll slightly back and the body shivers and she drops upon me, wet and her hair covers my face, and I lick the salt on her neck, and I think I will stay, but, again, the lights are flashing in the house of a coming storm and when Eva sits up, the face I see is being pulled back, as if she is slipping into the night, into the ink, her pale body the rim of memory, only to fade.

The lady looks into my eyes, slips off me, and curls at my side.

"James, you were here. You know you were."

"I felt so many known things rush through me, and then out again. When I try to fix on one it is gone, and I chase to another and it disappears, too."

"Try to remember our story. You were back just a moment ago, try to remember what my body brought back to you."

"I don't know our story. Maybe bits. The only thing I remember

63

for sure is Kurt and Vera. That summer of thunderstorms and the Impala in the sun and my body, young and lanky, brown. Then something happens, and there is blankness, an empty canvas stretching millions of miles long. I don't know. I hear something in me sometimes, a voice calling through deep, deep bone, but it never surfaces."

"I will tell you about me, James."

She is Eva Kapuscinski. She was a linguistics professor at the University of Warsaw. Her father was a partisan killed in that beguiling time of the 1950s, the beginning of the long run of communist tyranny; her mother was a poet who hanged herself from a tree when her verse turned less taut. Eva was raised in an orphanage; her skyline the ruins and smoke of a city rebuilding, years and years of rebuilding from a world war that, although ended much earlier, lingered over broken rooftops and cluttered rivers. She joined an underground Catholic church, took communion and prayed penances in back rooms and basements. She played soccer with the boys in the streets and later as a young woman at university she bought a bike with a basket, riding through the fog and drizzle to classes.

She was Eva, the girl with white roses and books on Mayan verbs and Yeats and Shakespeare. She took an assistant professorship at the university after graduation, comfortable in a cocoon of dissertations and classics, and secretly helped edit a newsletter for the resistance. The events from the outside passed under her desk lamp. It seemed that every day was capable of annihilation, the world's fate balanced on the tips of ICBMs and silos. Billions of people suspended, she thought, between the bear and that funny, long-legged man with the white beard and top hat the Americans called Uncle Sam. Mascots of freedom and doom; the world reduced to caricature.

One day, after securing tenure, Eva was approached about spying by a professor of mathematical theory, whom she had vaguely known from late-night university vodka parties. It was cleverly done, she thought; he spoke in equations, letters and numbers, so that he could be at once specific and obscure, and she could deduce what she wanted, accept or decline, and then each could go his or her way. She accepted, but not that night. It took a while, he with his equations, she with her texts. But they created a world of doublespeak, a place of secrets and codes right out in the open. They became lovers, but only in passing; spying Eva said was its own lover, demanding and jealous. She never knew exactly where her dispatches went, or how her syntax was parsed in a faraway office in Washington. She sent observations from the university, glimpses of life in the street, translations of articles she found interesting, and occasionally, after meeting them at a conference or university seminar, her thoughts on the communist politicians, so tight in their gray suits. Balloon men, she called them, fat and tense and tight, yet polished with the scrubbed pink skin of spas, except for the general in charge. He was pallid, a drab lanky gnome with a cigarette smile and black-circled eyes. She always had this fear that she'd be intercepted, unmasked; that men in long coats and tipped hats were watching her. It was hard to sleep and every creak and knock put a dreaded hollowness between the beats of her heart.

Then Gdansk. Such a harsh punch of a word. She could feel a change through the shipyards. It happened, gradually, at first, then broke like an ocean tide rushing out to sea. Posters and marchers and rain, the land trembling.

"That's how we met, James. The Berlin Wall fell, and you chased the echo. We met in a bar in Gdansk. The CIA didn't need my spying anymore. I needed a job. Remember? A guy from the Associated Press introduced us. I spoke five languages to you before you finished your beer. You looked at me, shook my hand, and said, 'Let's go.' I'll never forget that. So American. 'Let's go.' We went that night and you filed a story, and night after night you wrote stories as we traipsed across Europe, me on a fake French passport."

The lady in bed with me stops talking. She is crying on my shoulder. The room seems to have been through a storm. It is relaxed now. The lady has slipped to my chest, and I think she is sleeping, her breaths slow and long. I want to get up and step to the window, but I don't. I like the way she feels under my arm. I feel the length of her down my body. Stray clothes and towels lie rumpled on the floor. The light against the curtains is warm. It's the kind of light in a café in winter, enticing you to come in. I hear the waves. I study the lady's profile. Yes, I know her. I think. But she is evaporating from me; her story, like a movie, really, is dying too. Did I have such a life? I'm confused, but there is a body, a lady, alongside me, and even though I don't know all that I should, it feels good to feel another, to lie in a bed in a room like this.

I don't think I live here. I hear waves and footsteps down the hall, distant voices, the sound of metal, a sliding key, a door opening, closing, more footsteps, but softer, solitary, cross through the light beneath our door. The painting over the desk is of a schooner in a swelling sea, the crew is bracing against the wind, clinging to ropes in black slickers. A huge wave rises above the schooner. The men don't see it. They are facing the stern, battling other water. The scene is permanent, frozen in precise pencil and ink. The artist has left the crew's fate to the viewer. I think the captain will see the wave at the last minute, and the schooner will turn and plow head-on into it and come out the other side. Maybe.

What does Gdansk look like? If I was there I should know. If I wrote about a place, shouldn't something of it be stored in me? I slide farther down in the bed. The lady's face is next to mine on the pillow. Our noses touch. She sleeps pretty. I study her, but I do not know the things she wants me to know. I lift the covers a bit. Cool air rushes between our bodies. The lady doesn't stir. I peek into the tunnel cover and see us facing each other in our nakedness. I trace her breast with my finger. It is like another world, the light of the

66

room, barely penetrating the covers. It is a still life, only we are not posed or arranged. I smooth the covers flat and close my eyes. I hear the waves, the same sound as all those years ago when Kurt and Vera and I took that road trip to the beach and Vera hid from the man from Marrakesh.

nine

The man from Marrakesh. Yes, I know that story, too, or so it seems. But that phantom does not concern me now. I think of my half brother and Eva. James must be sleeping. Eva beside him. She loves James so much, the way we all want to be loved. But she is losing him. Losing means what is lost was once possessed. She's had that with James: the intimate rituals, the absences, the joy of reunion, the way a lover's face, a husband's face, is unexpectedly spotted on a sidewalk and for an instant he is a stranger bobbing in a crowd. But then the image claims itself and all is restored to what was. That is how the world should be, atoms and molecules, even if temporarily disrupted, falling into place, into patterns we mark, we remember. Into patterns we love.

When James tells me about Kurt and Vera, I tape him on a recorder hidden in my uniform. Not that I need to do it secretly; James wouldn't know or remember anyway. I feel like a spy, though. The thing is so small. I have hours of stories of Kurt and Vera. An oral history, I suppose. I listen to them on the bus on my way to work, although it's not really work to be with James. I listen to them in the bath and when I cook. I imagine I am in those stories, gliding in the Impala with them toward the beach, playing miniature golf with Kurt, rubbing lotion on Vera and trying on sunglasses and bathing suits with her while Kurt and my half brother Jim swim in the ocean. It was so grand in the time that it was good, in those days when the sun was bright and before the clouds rolled in, the way they do so unexpectedly, suddenly, over the beach.

I, too, went to the beach as a child, dove into the chilled waters and collected hermit crabs along the hard New England coast. I ate ice cream and felt sand between my toes and kissed my first boy behind a clam shack on the last day of August. We all have a summer love. But I didn't know I had another mother. I didn't know so much; yet despite this ignorance I grew. I became a voice in the universe, with sins and prayers, joys and redemptions, tuitions and leases, credit cards and memories. The scent of popcorn on sea air, cards clicking in bicycle spokes, a car alone on a highway in the snow, a drop of blood in underpants; scared, hurrying to the school nurse, who smiled, "You are a woman now." We change in years, days, hours, and seconds, but at some point invention stops and we become what we will die of. It is the in-betweens we seek: those thrilling moments when we stand apart and see the imprints that bear our name. I wonder about the first boy I kissed. Tyler Smart. Did he turn into a good man? Does he have a wife? Children? Does he remember me and my sunburned nose and the way I closed my eyes when he touched me?

I am dancing now, slow-dancing alone in James's room. I do this sometimes when the other night nurse goes on break. My mind wanders to music, my body drifts. I find it relaxing in the way I imagine people find repose in yoga or Valium or God. My brother's bed is made with clean linen, his pillow seems a new, white balloon. I dance around the bed and to the window. What must I look like from the street? The city is sleeping and no one sees, not even the moon hiding in clouds. I catch myself in the mirror, dark and white.

ten

The Beach Boys grew louder as the elevator dropped toward the lobby. Kurt hated the Beach Boys, said if that's what California was like he had no interest in ever going, and he'd never want to meet a girl like Barbara Ann; no, he was partial to the women who tormented Walter Jackson. The elevator doors opened and the girl at the front desk, the one whose cinnamon lip gloss I could still taste, winked at me and said: "Y'all have a nice evening, now."

"They're sure friendly down here," said Kurt. We stepped onto the boardwalk, the night breeze lifting Vera's dress. There was witch hazel and salt in the air, and a little bit of Kurt's Right Guard, but mostly the breeze was pure and refreshing. Vera ran a little ahead of us and twirled on the boardwalk, staring up at the moon and laughing and then running back to Kurt and hugging him, the two of them spinning, and people watching, not with angry or bemused stares, but with smiles that said, *Yes, on a night like this, with the moon big and white, that's what you do on Virginia Beach*.

"I want Howard Johnson's fried clams," said Kurt.

"No, Kurt. Not Howard Johnson's. Let's find a little hole-in-the-wall place with a one-eyed cook and fresh fish and . . ."

"We'll do the hole-in-the-wall place for breakfast, but right now I want some clams."

"They're not fresh, Kurt. They're frozen. It's not very exotic."

"I don't want exotic clams."

Vera looked at me and rolled her eyes. Kurt loved Howard Johnson's clams. When I was little, he'd throw me into the car and he and Mom and I would drive out of Philly and onto the Jersey Turnpike, up two exits to a rest stop with a big Howard Johnson's. Kurt would order a clam roll and a milk shake and sit there smiling, and my mom would ask, "Kurt, why are you so content with those clams?" Kurt said he didn't know. Maybe it was the booths and the low-hanging lights, and waitresses in custard-colored uniforms; maybe it was the ambience (an early dictionary word) of plates sliding under hot orange lights and chefs in tall hats; maybe it was the hiss and the steam and the coffee guys at the counter talking like they knew the world's secrets; maybe it was all that, but mostly he said the clams reminded him of being a boy, of getting dressed up and going out with his parents for that one special night a month. "You a boy now, Kurt?" Mom would tease.

"I am." He'd reach out and hold Mom's hand on the tabletop, his forearms cut and scraped from the shipyard, his hair damp from a shower.

"I don't see a HoJo's, Kurt."

"Right up here to the left at the bottom of this hotel. I asked that girl at the front desk."

"I'm not getting clams. I'll have a salad. But I'm sure the lettuce won't be fresh."

Kurt was not deterred by Vera's lack of enthusiasm. A hostess whose name tag said TINA led us to a booth by the window with a view of the ocean, breaking waves glowing in the distance and farther out silhouettes of fisherman casting in the pier lights. It was a great seat; it made you feel rich, not the money kind of rich, but the rich of being alive on a clear night in a window seat hovering over the boardwalk and watching the people below as if they're your own creations, and having a waitress named Debbie hand you a menu and lay out silverware.

"I don't need a menu," said Kurt.

Vera smiled. Kurt had won her over. HoJo's wasn't the Maghreb, but it was nice, Vera had to admit. She ordered a fruit bowl and a coffee. I chose a Monte Cristo sandwich. Kurt told the waitress he wanted not one but two little paper cups of tartar sauce for his clams; sometimes, he told Debbie, there's not enough. She agreed, made a note, and hurried off. Vera slid away from Kurt and moved closer to the window.

"Look at them all down there, walking and laughing, jumping to the sand and running to the water's edge. You ever wonder about all those people, all the people in the world you'll never meet? Could be a best friend down there you'll never have, a lover like no other. Just people and faces, really, but they make me wonder. You ever wonder about all those faces, Kurt?"

"I do. But right now I'm looking for Debbie's face and my clams."

"What about you, Jim?"

"Sometimes you think you know them."

Vera pushed her face closer to the window. She spoke to it, low and steady.

"I think there's a killer down there, waiting, hanging back in the darkness. I think that man from Marrakesh is here. I can feel him. When someone's been following you so long, you sense him; he becomes the twin you don't want. I bet he's out there, Jim, right now, looking up at us in this big lighted bird's nest."

She turned away from the window and slid back to Kurt.

"But he won't come tonight," she said, holding Kurt's hand and looking at me across the table. Kurt said nothing and stared ahead. I scanned the restaurant, looking for a man I thought might be from Marrakesh, but I had never seen anyone from Marrakesh before, so I looked for somebody suspicious. There was a guy sitting by himself at the end of the counter, but he was eating an ice cream cone, and a girl came over and took a lick, and I guessed he probably wasn't a killer, more likely the boyfriend of the waitress, but that was the thing about a killer, you never knew.

The food came and we ate in quiet. Kurt didn't enjoy his fried clams and two paper cups of tartar sauce the way he had hoped.

Vera excused herself. She was gone for a long time, and then we heard, from the outside, someone yelling, "Kurt, Kurt." We looked out the window and there was Vera standing on the boardwalk railing, holding three balloons and waving. Vera could do that, change a moment in a breath. She jumped into the sand and ran toward the waves, the balloons bobbing and disappearing in the darkness, until all we could see was Vera's white dress in the night. Kurt shook his head the way a man does when he reads something disturbing in the newspaper.

"C'mon, Jim. We better get down there."

"What should we do about this man she talks about?"

"I don't feel concerned yet. You scared?"

"I'm curious, and a little scared."

"That's two of us."

"He might have a gun."

Kurt looked at me and said nothing. I followed him to the beach. Vera danced in the surf.

"I let the balloons go and the night swallowed them, or they're still floating to the stars. I think they pop at a certain point."

"Atmospheric pressure," said Kurt.

"Aren't you a smart one."

"It's like in a plane when your ears pop."

"I thought you'd never been on a plane."

"I've read about it."

"The danger here has passed. I can feel it. Let's go win me a stuffed animal down the boardwalk."

"I'm good at pitching balls at milk bottles."

"Every man has his talent."

Kurt laughed. So did I. Vera ran out of the surf and held Kurt's hand. She put an arm around my shoulders. Her wet dress and cool skin brushed me; I felt the squeak of salt as she dried in the night. Kurt won Vera a lime-green alligator wearing a top hat.

It cost him four dollars and sixteen balls at a booth run by a man who wore a carpenter's nail sack for a change purse and had an accent from a history book. Vera liked him. He was exotic, not like HoJo's clams and 7-Eleven Slurpees. He told us he escaped from Hungary and moved in with an uncle in Chesapeake. "My country shit. Here better, but English is hard. Hungarian is not so difficult. I love Grand Funk Railroad." We walked on. Vera kissed Kurt and thanked him for the alligator. She named him Vlado. The world came to us through Vera. Hungary. Marrakesh. Vera said it was a world of spies and fragrances.

We walked back to the hotel. The girl at the front desk winked at me again. Kurt and Vera and I got in the elevator. Kurt put his fingers in his ears to block out the Beach Boys. I went to my room; Kurt and Vera rustled next door in 501, but then it quieted and I opened the balcony window to let in the sound of the waves. I kept the light off and turned on the TV. I flicked around and found an old black-and-white movie on a program called Fright Night. *Creature from the Black Lagoon.* It scared me when I was small, but now the creature was just a guy in a decorated wet suit with phony gills and big, unmoving, black bug eyes. I liked watching anyway, remembering the parts that once spooked me and wondering why I wasn't scared anymore. The Creature, a part of us but not, like the man from Hungary. Someone knocked. I guessed a killer from Marrakesh wouldn't be so polite, and when I creaked the door the girl from the front desk smiled and pushed her way in. She was a storm of cinnamon and perfume. She pasted her gum to the mirror, glossed her lips, and sat on the bed.

"Oh, I love this movie," she said. "That water's black like sin. The whole lagoon is evil."

"Seems fake."

"You're no fun. The creature's the devil."

"All monsters are the devil."

"Not all. Frankenstein wasn't the devil. He was body parts brought to life with lightning. I like that movie better than this one. When I'm alone at the front desk late at night, I make up scary movies in my head."

"Like what?"

"I was robbed once."

"In a movie."

"Real thing. A guy ran in with a knife and waved it in my face and told me to give him money. I handed him thirty-five dollars from the special 'robbery drawer' my daddy rigged up for the night shift. The big money we slide underneath in a second drawer with an electronic lock. The guy seemed startled when I gave him the money. He looked at it, looked at his knife, and ran out laughing down the boardwalk."

"You're lucky."

"You wanna smoke some pot?"

"I thought you were a Christian. A Baptist."

"I am, silly. But I'm a sinner, too. Not big sins, though." She laughed. "You can get saved again and again; my daddy says that's what he likes most about Jesus. The ability to fail."

She pulled out a small joint from her shorts pocket and lit it with a hotel match. She burned her fingers, her eyes watered, and she coughed. She hadn't smoked pot a lot, and neither had I. Twice, once in the rear parking lot at St. Jude's when I hoped the scent of it would mix in with the scent of incense and no one would notice, and the other time at the ball field around the corner from my house, sitting in the dark in a dugout with Scooter Meyers, listening to Elton John on a cassette player Scooter hauled around in a book bag. Most of the pot I saw was in tiny roaches in ashtrays of cars driven by longhairs just out of high school. Beer was bigger in my neighborhood. Six-packs on an autumn night, standing around flames in a barrel, guys talking about the Eagles' passing statistics and ward politics, looking at the stars and listening to fights and love echoing out of row houses, bits and pieces of lives slipping beyond brick walls and into the night, so everybody knew a little about everybody else, but not enough to pretend intimacy.

I didn't even drink a lot of beer. Maybe a bottle a week, if it was handed to me by a guy like Manny Jesus, whom everybody called Mr. Two-first-names, but not too loudly because Manny kept a silver Derringer tucked in his blue jeans. Kurt didn't drink a lot of beer, either, just that precious one after work on the stoop, and sometimes on a Friday night, he'd have a few extra, but not too many. On Sundays, he played tennis.

The girl handed me the joint.

"What's your name?"

"Jim."

"Yours?"

"Alice."

"That's an old person's name." I laughed.

"It is not. My daddy picked it when he saw a picture in the newspaper of the Bay Crab Queen the day I was born. Her name was Alice."

"What did your mom think about that?"

"She run off a week after she got out of the hospital with me. Took up with another man. Daddy was wrecked for months. That's when he found Jesus."

She took the joint back, pinching it in her fingers.

"It's Hawaiian or Colombian or something with a foreign name. My brother gets marijuana for waxing surfboards under the pier. He surfs, too. He's older. He went to Vietnam for a year, but my daddy says there's no soldier in him anymore."

She put the joint in the ashtray and went to the window and shushed the smoke out into the ocean breeze. She called me out to the balcony.

"Let the wind blow through you. It'll get rid of the pot smell."

We stood there awhile. She handed me a stick of gum and put more cinnamon gloss on her lips. She took my hand and said this is what it would be like when we got older, older and married with the kids sleeping in the house. Day's end and parents talking outside in the night. She wasn't speaking about being married to me; it was more general. She kissed me. It wasn't hard and fast like she had done hours earlier before I went out with Kurt and Vera to dinner. This time it was soft.

"I better git. My break's over and I gotta get back to the front desk."

She left the balcony and crossed the room, her blond hair thick down her tan back. She opened the door, smiled, and disappeared, the flash of her green halter the last of her I saw.

I was tired. The credits for the *Creature from the Black Lagoon* scrolled and the lady hosting Fright Night, a big-bosomed witch with an Eddie Munster hairdo, whom the guys back in Philly, and even Kurt, thought was sexy, announced that the next film would be the "creepy descent into madness when we enter the demented, demonic mind of perhaps our greatest horror actor, Vincent Price, in the classic *Pit and the Pendulum*."

I turned the TV off and lay on top of the bedcovers. The breeze was nice, the white curtain ghosting, and the scents of pot and cinnamon hanging around me. Alice was a strange girl. I was on a strange journey. My life in a bag and a suitcase, my dad next door with another strange girl, footsteps in the hallway, the crunch of the ice machine, footsteps returning, a key in a lock, the creak of a door, a laugh and surrender, the ocean tide changing, imperceptible, incremental, its wave lines rimmed by darting sandpipers pecking at crabs in the moonlight. I left the room and took the stairs down and out the back entrance to the beach. I mixed in with the mist and the night. Back in Philly, the *Inky* would be coming off the presses, the delivery trucks growling through the city and out to the suburbs. The paperboys would be waiting on their spider bikes in the dark, and the news would slap on doorways and driveways, slap, slap, slap, slap, hundreds of thousands of times before dawn.

I walked to a pier with no lights. It looked like ancient bones, a carcass in the darkness. I heard voices in the waves. A guy in a white T-shirt hopped up from a blanket and a girl sat up and tied her bathing suit top. I walked under the pier and cut over the beach to the boardwalk. Our hotel glowed with a few lights in the distance. I felt like a king in an old book, sneaking out of my castle and walking through my kingdom while my subjects slept. I imagined that's how God felt at night, looking down at the earth He made, quiet, the sinners and the missionaries sleeping, nobody doing anything wrong, nobody doing anything right, just the world spinning. A ball bounced across my feet and off the boardwalk, into the sand. A dog chased right behind it. An old guy in shorts, slippers, and an open bathrobe meandered out of an alley and onto the boardwalk.

"Crazy fucking dog I got. Never sleeps. Insomniac. I have to let him run for the next hour and maybe he'll drop. You got a dog out here?"

"Just me."

"Nice, huh. Not another soul around. It's how it is in winter. Just me and the dog, no tourists."

The dog scampered back and dropped the ball. The guy picked it up and hurled it down the boardwalk, the ball bouncing toward infinity, the dog in pursuit. The guy lifted a flask from his pocket. He sipped and we studied each other in the night. His face was gray-and-black stubble, but he had a good haircut and his robe, brocaded in gold stitching, was neat and clean, not the robe of a guy who might have wandered away from a state hospital. He capped the flask and lit a thin cigar. He was a writer. A technical writer. He wrote about science and medicine in journals and magazines. He was working on a story about a new mechanical heart valve that was smaller, thinner, and lighter than a dime. What was happening in laboratories was amazing; science was accelerating so fast that the world was being reborn in its own technology. He talked about grids and fiber optics and words flashing through this thing called ether. It sounded like science fiction. Even though it was real, it seemed fake, made up, and that was what enchanted him. Enchanted was his description. Putting words to such visions and inventions crowded him and he needed, with his dog, to escape his room and typewriter and wander the night and the beach thinking about star distances and cellular structures.

I asked him if he had ever been to Marrakesh. He hadn't. He knew about North Africa from maps and medical stories he wrote about parasites and waterborne diseases and how an epidemic becomes a pandemic and how it all can start with a microbe in a village nobody ever heard of. The guy made me think about the planet's many layers, so many sounds and silences coiling through deserts, jungles, and slums, like the one in Calcutta that Fr. Heaney took up Sunday collections for. You could never really know the world; you had to break it into the geographies that interested you most. He asked me what I wanted to do with my life. I told him that I'd like to see as much of the world as I could, even if I couldn't understand it all, it'd be nice to glimpse with my own eyes. He stood with his cigar and looked at the black ocean.

"Make sure you see it," he said. "It's changing fast, not like evolution. That's a slow and grinding dance. But today there's something new with every rotation. A new medicine, a new disease, a new way to heal a wound, a new weapon to kill with. The human capacity to at once save itself and annihilate itself amazes me. Truly amazes me. I live in the science of it."

"You have a family?"

"Just that dog and my typewriter. I had a wife. She died in a plane crash. Ice on the wing. They have new systems and chemical solutions now to de-ice planes."

"My mom died, too. She was hit by a car that skidded on ice."

"Frozen water. Pretty, but dangerous. I'm sorry about that."

"I miss her."

The guy sipped from his flask. His dog returned, panting, and dropped the ball. The guy picked it up and he and the dog walked back toward the alley. He turned and gave one of those two-finger waves off the eyebrow, the kind in the Bogart movies. The air changed; pink and orange needles brightened the gray horizon, but it was still night on the boardwalk, as if the dawn were sneaking in on the darkness, starting from way out, and slowly, the way you turn a kaleidoscope, bleeding the sky with color.

I walked back to the hotel. Alice was sleeping at the front desk, her head on her arm, her Bible open. I took the stairs and slipped into 503. The scent of pot was gone and the room was sticky, a salt film on the mirror, and sitting in the corner, though I didn't notice at first, was Vera, holding a silver pistol in her hand with her purse on her lap.

"I knocked but you weren't here. These locks are easy to pick. He's here, Jim. I saw him again. Out there, on the beach. I was on the balcony while Kurt was sleeping, and there he was standing under the boardwalk light, looking up at me. We gotta get out of here, Jim. As soon as Kurt wakes up.

"I don't want you to worry. He doesn't want you. Only me. That's why I have this. It's a thirty-eight caliber. I don't know much about guns but the man who sold it to me said it was the kind of gun for what I needed."

"Does Kurt know you have a gun?"

"I've kept it hidden. You don't pull a gun out when you first meet a man. Don't worry, it'll be all right. But this guy keeps coming, following me like a stink or a shadow and I don't know why he just won't let me be. Why he won't let that time go, believing he could bring the Maghreb here. Go to the balcony, Jim. See if he's still there."

There was no one under the boardwalk light, just a few circling seagulls. I wondered if it was the same guy I had seen hours earlier.

"Vera, I think you should put the gun away. There's no one out there right now."

"I've been sitting here for two hours, frozen, hunched in this corner. I can't hold this gun much longer anyway. Here, Jim, take it and put it in my purse."

I stepped toward her and took the pistol. It was dense and as heavy as a paperweight. I put it in her purse and lay the purse on the bed. Vera stood and hugged me; she hugged me hard, so hard I could feel beneath her skin into the core of her and it reminded me of that Bible passage "I can count all my bones." Vera pulled back and looked at me and hugged me again. She laughed and cried in my ear.

"Look at us, Jim, in this room above the ocean, hiding; we are hiding from a crazy man speaking another language. It's like a storybook. But we won't let him get us. We won't let him. We'll get Kurt, get the Impala and go. We'll shake him, Jim. This time we'll shake him for good."

She sat on the bed, still for a few minutes, then slumped over and curled up like a sea horse.

"Jim, I'm going to sleep for an hour or so. Keep watch."

I sat in the chair. Vera's breathing slowed. I lifted her purse, a big, rattling macramé sack; the gun slipped to the bottom. I peeked and reached in and felt sand and lipstick and lighters and bobby pins and loose tobacco and papers and three vials for pills, all empty. There was a postcard by Edward Hopper and a map drawn on the back of an envelope. It was our hotel and the boardwalk and the streets and alleys around it and the road to the interstate and a star where the

Impala was parked. There were arrows on the streets, each leading through twists and turns to the interstate. Beneath the map it read: "Escape route. Wait till last minute. Keep clothes ready. Go quickly. Keep Kurt and Jim close, so don't have to be looked for. Running out of time, energy."

Vera's purse was full of escape maps. There was a map of our neighborhood in Philly, and another one from around the tennis court where Kurt played that guy on the Eastern Shore, and a few more from places I didn't recognize. There was a black-and-white picture of a girl in a snowsuit sitting by a swing set, with sledders in the distance; another picture of the same girl running on a grassy hill in a summer dress. There were no dates, but you could tell they were long-ago photographs, the kind Kurt kept in a shoe box from his boyhood. They didn't give enough clues, like clothes or cars or obvious things, to place a time. The images were faint, nearly lifeless, like pictures of Civil War generals sitting around tents. The little girl in the pictures had dark hair and fair skin and must have been Vera, but I couldn't tell.

I dropped the pictures into the purse and pulled out a letter. It was written by Vera and mailed to the same Cleveland address it was sent from. I opened the envelope:

> To whom it may concern. As I'm writing this, I can see him through the white curtains on the corner. He's smoking a cigarette, reading the paper at the bus stop. Why does he keep following me? Never to rest. When night comes, I'll mail this letter. If I escape him, you will never read it. I have sent it to my apartment, and if I receive it here in a few days, it means I have survived. If not, it will come into your hands when in days, weeks, or maybe months someone discovers I am missing. My plan is to leave here next week. I am already packed. I am looking for safety. Is there such a thing? Look

at him out there. Can't they see he is different, this man from
Marrakesh? His skin, his mood, his shoes, all different and
dangerous. But people don't see the danger he is. Look at
the man standing next to him. Smiling and talking to him
over their newspapers. He fools everyone so well. His accent.
So smooth. It lures you in, a trick, a ploy, and then it's too
late. He's even fooled the police. I bought a gun. I loaded it.
Don't know how to use it, but I feel better, the weight of it
makes me feel better. I'm doing something. Not a victim. I
must mail this. I hope you don't receive this letter. If you do,
on the next page is a drawing and the name of the man who
murdered me. Sincerely, Vera.

I turned the page and looked at the pencil-and-ink man Vera
had drawn: hair tapered close to his head, eyes far apart, a nose, not
broad, but not angular, either, his chin hiding in the scarf wrapped
around his neck. I didn't know if I'd recognize him if I passed him
on the boardwalk, although there was a scar shaped like a diamond
on his cheek. Mounir. No last name. I put the letter and drawing
back and closed the purse. I didn't want to know more.

I looked at Vera, sleeping. I sat on the floor by the bed and studied
her. She was big in waking life, a force pulling you into her, like the
way in Philly when she slid into the diner booth and started chattering to Kurt and me. You had to listen; the words whirled, came at
you with stories of all the things you didn't know, and the things you
wanted to know, the things you knew were out there half sketched,
but Vera filled them in, gave them the feel of steel. The souks, Cairo,
trinkets in Bedouin hands, desert treks to the sea. But sleeping, Vera
was small, thin, her hair mussed and dull, all her energy vanished.

I wished there was a record player in the room. I felt like listening
to the Beatles' *White Album,* real soft, especially "Dear Prudence"
and "Julia." I missed my music. Kurt and Vera and I shared what

was on the radio, but to me music was private; it was as personal as secrets, even more part of you than the sins you whispered at confession. I wanted to put the needle on the groove, to hear the crackle and scratch and then John Lennon singing about the mother he had lost. I went to the window. I wanted to see the man from Marrakesh on the boardwalk. I wanted him to wave to me. I wanted to know he was there, that he was more than pencil and ink. You can't have demons scratching at the edges all the time; they have to climb aboard and show themselves just like the monster in the *Creature from the Black Lagoon* did. Maybe the man from Marrakesh was a killer, was all the things Vera was so spooked about, but I needed to see him. Every time Kurt and I looked he was gone. He could have been clever, real clever, like Vera said, a jinn possessed of special powers from the Maghreb. Not science-fiction weirdo powers, but powers and auras people have from living in deserts and mountains. I looked down. Nothing, except two joggers, a man and a woman, talking and looking at each other as they panted down the boardwalk.

I left Vera sleeping and went to Room 501. I checked the door. It was open and through the white curtain I saw Kurt sitting on the balcony, his shirt off, his hair slicked back from a shower, the scents of talcum and Right Guard in the room. He had his eyes closed and face toward the sun.

"Vera's next door," I said.

"I know."

"She's got a gun."

"I know. I took the bullets out back in Maryland."

The morning breeze was cool, but you could feel threads of heat in it like when you jumped into the ocean and a warm current snaked past you.

"What should we do?"

"I don't know, Jim. It was like an adventure back in Philly. This woman comes out of the night and changes things for us, telling us about places, bringing us colors and sounds and smells, hitting tennis balls in the alley. It was different and that's what I wanted for a while. No gray paint in the shipyard. No wife and mother buried in the earth. I miss her, Jim. I had to get away from all the things, the tiniest damn things that brought her back into that house making me think she was in the kitchen or running a bath upstairs. You know what I mean? Did you feel it, too? She was there but we couldn't have her."

"I thought sometimes I heard her in the backroom listening to the radio and painting her watercolors. Remember what she said after taking that painting class at the Y?"

"Seep and bleed."

"Yeah, let the colors 'seep and bleed across the canvas.'"

"I think she only finished one."

"The rowers on the river."

Kurt kept his eyes on the waves and the empty beach. He was done talking about Mom. I saw it in the way his jaw tightened. He was tan and built hard, his muscles sturdy and long like dock rope, but they fit his lean frame. He didn't seem a father. He was a man on a balcony, sun and breeze on his face, all his logic and the things he knew, all those traits a son sees in his father from a distance, were loosened, and up close Kurt was a man wanting to be rearranged back to what he was before. I thought it must be hard for a father to be caught between the two sides of himself. I felt split, too. But it was different; my history was brief, too young to be a record, grooved and set with rhythms.

"Is there a guy from Marrakesh? I did see a man under the board-walk light last night, but he didn't look like someone to be scared of."

"I'm not certain about any of this, Jim. Should we go to the cops? And say what? I don't know if I believe Vera or not, but I wouldn't feel right abandoning her. I can't get into that Impala and leave. I guess in this short time she's become part of us. Not like Mom, but somebody who has filled in some of the blank spaces. It's only right to protect her from whatever scares her. But what if this man is really out there? Am I putting us in too much danger?"

I didn't know, either, so I sat with Kurt on the balcony, saying nothing, listening to the morning waves.

spinning in a jagged yellow circle just out of reach. The man reminds me of something, but I can't think what. I feel like I'm rapping at a door that won't open; the lady beside me has her arm around me and her head on my shoulder and we're walking as if this is how it should be, but I don't know how it should be.

"Here we are, James. The diner, remember? Best pancakes in the world, you say. I don't like them."

Bells ring over the door. We slip into a booth. A waitress with a pot flips over two cups and pours before I get out of my coat. She drops two creams in front of me and spins away. It is fast in here, crowded with smoke and people, the scent of syrup and breaking eggs, the sizzle and the sound of a whisk through batter. The cook, a man peeking from a cutout window, like a prisoner in a steamy cell, yells at the waitress and she yells back, "Hash browns, hash browns, twice. For God sakes it's always hash browns. You think someone's gonna order something different?"

She walks over to the lady and me.

"What'll ya have?"

"Pancakes."

"Short or tall?"

I cock my head.

"Stack, short or tall?"

The lady says short. With orange juice and extra butter.

"You?"

"Coffee. Toast and jam."

The lady sitting across from me takes my hand and gets up and steps toward me, combing my hair with her fingers. "Your hair, James, always wild. A mind of its own."

She sits back down.

"Do you want to hear more stories about yourself, about us?"

She pulls a fat envelope from her bag and lays it on the table. The pancakes and syrup come. The table is set with juice and coffee and sliced toast. It is neat, inviting, a simple thing, but it makes me feel connected, rooted in certainty. I close my eyes. All black, except this bright space, like a lone star in a night sky. Kurt and Vera. I open my eyes, stare at the lady in front of me, and quickly close my eyes, hoping to see an image of her rise in the blackness, but nothing comes, only Kurt and Vera. There must be more, but I can't say for sure. But I do know things. I know the beach, the waves, the wind. The elements. I know what it means when a man juggles lemons and a boy watches; I know, I see all things outside of me, the real world, I guess, but I don't know where I fit in. I am a murdered man drawn in chalk on the sidewalk, contours and emptiness. The lady whispers through the rattle of cups and sliding plates.

"We were on holiday outside Tunis," she begins. "We needed a break from Europe and its post-Soviet commotion. It was three years after we met, 1992. We had married a year earlier, just two weeks before you went to Iraq for the first Gulf war. Not much of a war, was it, James? 'Fires in the desert,' you said, 'sirens and sand in the hotels.' But in '92 we rented a whitewashed bungalow on the beach. We sailed in the mornings and swam and slept in the afternoons. It was how vacations should be, James. Just weather and waves on your soul, nothing else. Do you need more syrup?"

"No, thank you."

"Tunis, near Carthage along the cliffs. You don't remember, James, and that is such a shame, such a pity not to remember what so few people see. We had planned to go to Marrakesh."

She looks at me.

"Ahh, I see Marrakesh sparks a memory."

"Vera told me about Marrakesh. I was a boy. She said I had to go to Marrakesh, but there was a man . . ."

"Yes, James. I know, but we never made it to Marrakesh. Do you remember?"

"I don't remember anything. You give me a strand of something that supposedly happened in another time, in another place. But what do I do with it? Do you understand? I don't know."

"Don't be angry."

The lady sips her coffee, spreads blueberry jam on toast.

"I was pregnant. That's why we didn't get to Marrakesh. I was only a few months, the time when the body changes like a little science project. Blue veins and a thicker belly. We hadn't told anyone. We wanted it, James. For some reason, despite our wandering lives, we wanted a child."

She leans forward.

"Late one night on the beach the pain came. We took a taxi. I remember leaning back looking at the moon in the rear window. It was yellow and white. Big, like a planet that had slipped its orbit and was drifting toward us. Beautiful. The streets and alleys we drove through and all the people we passed, all going about their lives on a warm evening, all of them not knowing about us, who we were or what we were losing. Blood in the taxi and on my hands and on your clothes. I fell away.

"When I awoke I saw you at the foot of the bed, a ceiling fan spinning slowly above you. I remember that image so distinctly. The whole room. The white linen, the heavy, chipped metal bed, the IV, the nurse in her strangely folded hat. I knew that the unborn baby that left me took something with it. I could have no more children. I felt it before you said it. You held my hand through the night and I thought that my body, my insides were like the Sahara in southern Egypt with its sharp rocks and painted caves. Arid yet beguiling. You didn't like that metaphor. You said it was too easy. Too biblical, the desert barrenness, using geography like shorthand. But you, for once, had no metaphor of your own, so I hung on to mine for a while, a long while, James."

She sips her coffee.

"We stayed in the bungalow for a few days, until the bleeding stopped. We flew to Paris, but Paris wasn't the same. Nothing was the same, not for a while. Days and hours. Every spoken word leading back to that night of the big moon. It eased over time. We made love again and there were new stories to write, and James, it was our love, our love that saved us. That sounds trite, I know, but that doesn't make it any less true. But our lost baby was there, and sometimes, late at night, each of us would feel it, a slight prick that by morning would pass."

"Did we want a boy or a girl?"

"We didn't care. We didn't know."

"Was there a funeral?"

"No. I was only a few months' pregnant, James. There was nothing."

"There was something."

"Yes . . ."

The lady who says she's my wife is now crying over her coffee and toast. It is a slow cry, the kind that causes no disturbance. I was to be a father, like Kurt. I don't remember Tunis, the hospital, the way she said she bled. How can a man have blood on his clothes, the blood of his child, and not remember? She wipes her eyes and takes my hand.

"That story is not in this big envelope of your clippings I carry. It never appeared in a newspaper. It's our private story, James. I tell it to you each time I see you, hoping. It's like a part of a play I have rehearsed. But it is not rote. It is never rote. It feels as if it's new in each telling. I cry each time. Each time it's so real to me. And all I want you to say is, *Yes, Eva. I remember.* Just that. A feeling that you carry it, too, that no matter what's happening in your brain, there's a tissue, something in you, that holds that memory, a memory deeper than thought. I'm silly and rambling, James, and it's useless. I'm talking to a man with a blank face."

She smears jam on her toast, puts the knife down hard. She leans toward me.

"I'm angry that this story has become mine alone. My burden, not yours. That's not fair, James. Part of me thinks part of you is blessed not to know that story. Is that selfish?"

She leans back and picks up the knife, studies the jam on its blade; she seems to bury a word, or maybe a sentence, behind her lips. She breathes out, closes, then slowly opens, her eyes.

"My anger, you forgot my anger," she says, smiling, but not really happy. "Did you even know I was angry two seconds ago? What an ideal marriage we have, James. You don't hold my sins against me."

The waitress pours coffee. The lady eats her toast. Blueberry stains her teeth, but she doesn't care. I like her. I want to remember her. We pay the bill and stroll (a funny word) on the boardwalk; the sun turns the ocean into a bright mirror and the waves have no fury; they droop onto the beach in lazy curls. The amusement park. The clown face, the bumper cars, the Ferris wheel, the twirling teacups, the House of Horrors, the merry-go-round all quiet, cold and quiet, glazed in the salt spray of the ocean. We sit. The lady slips an arm through mine.

"We talked about this years ago, James. This kind of moment of sitting along this beach after all our travels. To have a house down the block with a wraparound porch and big windows. You in one, writing books; me in the other, translating documents and files for the UN. That's what I do now, James. But I live in New York, in a small apartment with a stunning view of the river, but no wraparound. We lived there together, but when you started slipping the doctors thought it'd be best to bring you back to Philly. They have the best care for your sort of problem. Maybe, they said, the streets and neighborhoods of your childhood would awaken memories beyond just Kurt and Vera. You remember your street, don't you?"

"Clare Street. Fourteen-thirteen Clare Street. About midway down the block. The McMurphys on one side. The Kowalskys on the other. I know all that like yesterday. Fr. Heaney in his rectory window, reading murder mysteries and hearing confessions. That's what I know. Kurt and Vera. That time. Like yesterday."

"The beach is best like this. We used to make up games. We'd sit on this very bench in autumn. Nobody but us. We'd make up stories about marooned galleons and pirates. You'd start them and I'd add on and we'd switch the story back and forth, building it for hours."

"I like it here. I like the stillness. Can we sit for a while?"

"As long as you like. Look what I have."

She reaches into her big purse. "Vranac."

"Wine?"

"Yes, James. It used to be your favorite. Sometimes when you drink it, you remember things. I forgot glasses, though. We'll have to drink from the bottle."

"Like winos. In Philly, we had winos."

"We had them in Poland, too. But there they drank vodka and peed on the sides of buildings and froze to death in winter."

"You're from Poland?"

"A long time ago. I live in New York now."

"Is it too early to drink wine?"

"Time doesn't matter, does it?"

She rubs her hand over mine.

"You wrote a story on wine in Tuscany. We went from vineyard to vineyard, sampling, learning about the sun, the soil, the minerals. Quite an alchemy. And the Italians, 'quote machines,' you called them. The vineyard owners spoke for hours about land and harvest. So many things conspiring in the air and in the dirt to make a magnificent wine or a wondrous failure."

The lady uncorks the wine and hands me the bottle, and for a second I think I remember something, but then I don't. I look at the sea. The sun is behind us, the clouds low. Winter is coming. I like this wine.

"Let's talk about news, James. Today's news. Big change in the world again. A black man is running for president. His name is Barack Obama. He is eloquent, James. Eloquent the way leaders should be, not like most of them today. There is no grandeur in them. No romance. No dreams, like the dreams we had when the Wall fell. You should be there, writing about all this."

"Nixon."

"Nixon?"

"I remember Nixon. Those hearings in 1972, or was it '73. Kurt said Nixon skulked. Kurt didn't like politicians. He said Democrat or Republican, they were destined to disappoint. I like that word. Skulked."

"He was a skulker, yes. He's dead, James. A while now."

"He used to be president. Watergate."

"The one now is worse than Nixon. Bush."

"Bush?"

"He's a twit. He comes to the UN sometimes. He speaks English, but you wouldn't know. Other translators tell me they can't fit his syntax and imagery into their languages. He should be in jail."

"That bad?"

"Worse."

The lady takes another sip of wine. She hands me the bottle and puts her head on my shoulder. A man with fishing poles and a tin bucket walks past; a woman follows with two folding chairs. They descend the boardwalk steps to the beach. He's heavyset with a ball cap and a windbreaker and green boots up to his knees. He is unsteady in the sand, favoring his left knee. The woman wears a ball cap, too; blue jeans, a big sweatshirt and long knitted scarf that snakes in the wind. The woman unfolds the chair. The man casts a line into the surf and hands the pole to the woman; he casts a second one and holds it himself and sits down next to her at the rim of the beach break. He kisses her on the cheek. They sit, two shadows in the sun, water misting around them, their chairs slightly sinking in the sand.

A man clatters down the boardwalk with a guitar. He stops and sits on the bench next to the lady next to me. The man strums and sings — his voice a ragged cough of words — of melting ice caps, butchered trees, dying rain forests, pollution, smog, warming oceans, Venice sinking, "a world gone mad, slipping from the palms of God." He rolls his eyebrows and stands. "I'm just a messenger," he says, spinning away in wide slow circles, a strange planet in a tattered coat.

We watch, until she laughs, takes the bottle from me, and sips. The lady rises. She kisses me on the forehead, brushes my hair with her fingers.

"A wild sea, that hair."

It feels good. The ocean. The wind. The lady's fingers on my scalp, so brief. She sits and pulls an envelope from her bag. She unfolds a newspaper clipping; it rattles in the wind. The headline: MEMORY KEPT ALIVE, BRICK BY BRICK.

Walter Schmidt lived in Dusseldorf. He memorialized Jews killed in the Holocaust by painting their names on bricks across the city. The police told him to stop, but he wouldn't; he went from neighborhood to neighborhood. His mission was to paint six million names. He was up to 726,000. He carried a thin sable brush and a small can of white paint in his valise. He was demure, whispery-voiced, dressed like a banker, a man you wouldn't suspect of defacing property. He said: "We have atoned. Oh God, we have atoned, but we haven't suffered to the extent of our victims. That is the paradox. We atone with sorrow that can never be as deep as the horror. This bothers me."

The man lived with his wife and drove a subway train from dawn until two in the afternoon. He'd come home, change into a suit, and head back out to paint names until dusk; each brick, a tiny tombstone. He was occasionally beaten up by neo-Nazis, but the city came to know and admire his strange, fastidious mission, although, when some heard he was in their street, they stood guard over their homes and bricks. He said, "When you write your newspaper story, just use the names, one name strung after the other. Imagine the impact of names, but no other words. Don't you think that would be powerful? Just names. Imagination can fill in the rest. That would be a story people would remember."

He went to the same pub every day after his painting was done. He'd wash his face, clean his brush in the sink, comb his hair, and drink one beer alone before going home to his wife. "I won't get to all the names before I die," he said. "Isn't that something?"

The lady says, "I liked that man the best, James. Of all the interviews we did over all those years, I liked that little man from Dusseldorf the best."

"I don't remember."

"I know, but you were there, whether you remember or not."

"It's cold."

"Should we go?"

"Let's sit a little longer. I'm cold but I like it here."

"This used to be one of your favorite places. Right here on this bench."

"I can imagine. I do like it here. It makes me think of Kurt and Vera and the man from Marrakesh."

twelve

Eva called. She's going to keep James at the Jersey Shore another day. There was a brief moment when he came back and remembered her. Eva says there must be some way to hold that, to keep it centered, like the air bubble in a mason's level. I think not. That flash of memory is incandescent, but not sustainable. I have heard enough doctors, read enough charts, changed enough diapers of confused men who can't remember where or how to shit. James is headed there, maybe not for a while, but that is his slope. I like to think of miracles, though. Maybe. Perhaps. I'd like James to know me, not just as the woman in white, but as his half sister, the daughter of Kurt and Vera. Will I ever tell him? I don't know. He wouldn't remember for more than a fleeting moment, anyway.

I was conceived in Virginia Beach. This is what Vera told me in her letter. She said she felt the moment it happened. The moon luring the tide, the waves distant. It's a pretty way to be made. "A glorious conception," she wrote. The letter came to me quite unexpectedly. The way things do, like hurricanes, wars, and tsunamis that whirl in out of nowhere and make us rebuild. The letter was yellow and worn. I unfolded it, pressed my face against its pages, and breathed in Vera, but there was no scent of her, only old air and old paper and the cursive strokes of her desperate life. I was working as a nurse in Boston at the time — strange fate that I should have chosen the profession my half brother so needs. I had no husband, no children. I was dating a botanist. We took excursions into gardens and forests and graveyards. He could identify the mosses growing in tiny blooms on the tombstones of those who fought in the Revolution. His name was Jacob Myerson. We still see each other occasionally, but now that I've moved to Philadelphia to be near James, not as often. Jacob doesn't know about James. I told him I left Boston for a more challenging job. He believed me. When Jacob visits we walk the trails along the river and with an envelope and tweezers, he collects vegetation. Like me, he is meticulous; we have intense conversations about pollination, rain forests, savannas, and how trees store carbon dioxide deep in their cores. He fears the world is slowly dying. I tell him about hearts and veins and minds. We go to movies — mostly documentaries in foreign languages — and walk along South Street, window-shopping and listening to music rolling from doorways into the night. We eat pizza and drink cream soda along the water, and in the distance I see the gray hulks of old navy ships and their big white numbers, their strung lights pretty as stars. We return to my place with a bottle of wine and have sex; afterward, while Jacob sleeps, I trace the muscles of his body and think of the shore and the way waves crash against the pier and what it would have been like to have been born Chinese or Iranian. On Sunday mornings, Jacob rises early, leaves a pressed flower near the coffeemaker, and disappears out the door to the train that will carry him home to Boston. It's a nice arrangement, shy of fulfilling, but then again not overbearing. I go jogging on those mornings. I am swift and lithe, always have been, even at this age when the knees need more coaxing than they once did. Through the peal of church bells, I run across Rittenhouse Square, past cut flowers, jars of apple butter, and bundles of newspapers; I glide through colonial streets, beyond men selling black felt triangle hats and Ben Franklin spectacles; I slip through history, breathing in oil and distant ocean, turning through alleys the sun has yet to reach; I push on, sweat on my brow, my legs rhythmic as pistons; I run with no music in my ears except the sound of my footsteps against the waking city; I whisk past the gleam and smoke of diners to the quiet warehouses on the outskirts; I think of Vera and Kurt, young and alive, falling in love, spirits and ghosts denied me; I run until I weep. I let the tears fall. It feels good to let them fall. I am my own mystery, an incomplete daughter, an unknown sister. After a few minutes, I turn, look back over the miles I have come, and begin the journey home.

James was easy to find. I typed his name in Google. It was like a research project on a plant, a name, a being I never knew existed, but was related to, growing out there in the world. There were seventy-three pages of hits on James. He was a journalist, but then, suddenly, he vanished. I called his old paper and tracked him to this nursing-home/convalescent-center/rehab-facility/or-any-other-name-that-makes-you-feel-comfortable-about-a-place-that-cares-for-those-losing-their-marbles.

James looks just like my father, Kurt. Vera left me a picture of her and Kurt; it's black and white and was taken, I think, in one of those booths with a sliding curtain that are so popular at catching moments that don't last beyond the beach. James doesn't know me, but he is blood. The microscopic cells coursing through him are similar in patterns to mine. I think you need to know the person who is your blood. I never had that, and it's funny, ironic, I guess, that the only person connected to me by molecular structures is a man who doesn't know who I am from one day to the next.

I crave the memory he is losing.

I love it when he talks about my parents during that summer at the beach. But James's stories don't go all the way to the end when things turned nasty. And even hearing them, beautiful as they are, they are not flesh and bone; they cannot be caressed, whispered to; they cannot give a daughter, a sister, the touch, the warmth she needs. But they are all I have, words and words and words, stored and living in my mind.

What is in me? So many intricacies I do not know. Am I bound for a void like James? Or confusion like my mother? Was she confused? Or did she just see things others couldn't? There are too many spaces between the lines, and perhaps something is hiding in me, a deformity of spirit or an odd permutation of cell. A voice yet unheard.

The sky outside James's window fills with strands of blowing ash, thousands, maybe millions of them, twirling and swimming like slender black fish out of a sea of smoke rising from a fire at the city's edge. A landfill? A refinery? The fire glows and mixes with the dusk. I watch. The smoke fattens; the ash shifts with the wind, toward James's window, then away, then back again.

thirteen

Kurt and I went back into my room. Vera was still sleeping, her macramé purse, the one with the gun in it, lay beside her on the bed. Kurt went to the mirror and studied himself. He rubbed his hands under his eyes and through his hair.

"I found a gray one the other day, Jim. On my temple like a silver thread. The sunlight caught it when I was shaving. At first I thought it was paint from the shipyard."

I stepped to the mirror.

"Where?"

"I yanked it out."

"It'll come back."

"Nah, I got the root and all."

"It's pigment. We learned it in biology class. Your body's losing its color. Sister Hanrahan says the body's more complicated than the universe."

"When'd you get so smart?"

I shrugged. "Simple biology."

Even though we were whispering, Vera stirred. She rolled over, curling around her purse, drooling like a child, at peace.

"Should we wake her?"

"Let her sleep a little more. I don't think she's slept much in days. Let's go for a swim. I'll write her a note."

"What about the gun?"

"I told you I took the bullets out."

"What if she wakes and sees the man from Marrakesh."

"She doesn't usually see him in the mornings. C'mon let's swim."

The beach was quiet. It was too early for day-trippers. Kurt sprinted toward the water and dove, a spear cutting through a wave and rising beyond. He stood and shook the water out of his hair and dove again. I followed. The ocean was cold, sharp, stinging my sunburn. Kurt jumped on me; he wrestled and lifted me and threw me into a wave, and when I surfaced he did it again, and he kept laughing.

"When you were small I could throw you a mile."

Another wave came and knocked us both down. The undertow pulled at my calves.

"Let's get past these waves to deeper water."

Kurt didn't swim like he played tennis. On the tennis court, he was compact, quick, precise; every movement a burst. But in the water, he seemed big and languid, moving with a long crawl through the currents like a steamship. We were about seventy yards offshore, at the place where the water gathers just before it rises and rolls toward land. It was peaceful out there. My body lifted and dipped and I felt as if I were on a slow-motion roller coaster, a bobbing speck in what the Indians in this area once called "the Great Water." The Indians were gone but there was a brochure in the hotel lobby advertising Indian tours and an Indian museum. The Indians pictured in the brochure didn't look like Indians, though. Their skin was the orangey color of an indoor tan and their wigs and suede clothes looked as if pulled from a Halloween box; they seemed like dressed-up car salesman and undertakers standing around a tepee and a fake fire.

The water rose; I ascended. I was glad to be out here alone with Kurt. All sounds gone except our breaths, our words, our hands treading water, the currents below us running like icy slivers around my ankles.

"I wonder what we look like to a fish."

"Weird."

"Sometimes at the shipyard a school of fish swims in. I think they get lost and take a wrong turn where the ocean meets the river. They come up along the ships. You can see they're panicked and want to escape to the sea. Their white bellies flash in the rusty water. They splash and suddenly it all goes silent and the water calms and you can see them skimming beneath the surface heading back to the wide water as if one of them had found the way and was leading the others. They look like a dark cloud of bees, moving fast through the jetty.

"You tired, Jim?"

"Not yet."

"It's nice, isn't it?"

"Changes your perspective."

"I'm going to have to take that dictionary away from you. Pigment. Perspective. You must have worked your way up to the P's."

"I jump around so it's more interesting."

Kurt stopped treading water and floated on his back. I did the same. My ears immersed, I heard only the pulse of the depths, but every now and then, when I'd lift with a gathering wave, my ears broke the surface and I'd hear, for a split second, the cry of a seagull or a kid shrieking on the beach. When my ears went back under, the moan of the deep returned with the sound of my beating heart. I heard my body from the inside, a fleshy machine doing its work, like a car hood sprung open in an alley garage, belts and pistons humming like music.

I thought about Alice, the girl at the front desk with cinnamon lip gloss and halter tops. She kissed me softly the other night. I liked that; there was no rush and I heard her breathe and I listened to the breeze on the balcony and a muted scream from the *Creature from the Black Lagoon* on the TV. What would happen to Alice? Would she become queen of the Crab Festival like her Baptist daddy wanted? Or maybe she'd just get old and fill out the hotel ledger page after page, year after year, smiling to vacationers and handing keys to her splay-footed uncle, the ancient, slumped bellboy with the stained jacket. How many other boys and men would she kiss? How many halter tops did she own? How many girls would I kiss? Would I learn all the words there were to know?

I felt like a slip of paper floating beneath the sun, my body bending and rippling with the water. What if I drifted out to sea like Kurt's fish racing beyond the jetty, past freighters and sharks to a new beach in another part of the world? I was weightless, my body like a jellyfish left to the ocean's whim. I felt out of my skin, my skin had become the cool water.

My thoughts ran. I liked John Lennon better than Paul McCartney, but Paul had a better voice for harmony; John's was more wiry, built less for unison than for wit; others would disagree, believing that John and Paul were as harmonic as Simon and Garfunkel. Could I love a girl forever? Kurt would have loved Mom that long. The universe was ever expanding, unfolding in gases, black holes, and constellations. I loved looking through the telescope Nut Johnson kept on his roof in Philly. We'd go up on winter nights; the sky hard and black as an eight ball, and through our little clouds of breath we'd see pricks of light, swirls of white, and, if we were lucky, comets shooting like ice balls fired from cannons. We'd aim at Mrs. Romano's bedroom window and study her silhouette in the pulled shade, the telescope sharpening her features so that as she undressed, and if she were turned to the side, you could see her hair tumble out of the tight bun she wore; you could see her nipples rise. Nut called her nipples splendid. On some nights, Mr. Romano would come into the room and the light would go off and the shade would go blank and Nut and I would look at each other and smile, and Nut would say, "I'd love to be Mr. Romano." We'd zero in on Fr. Heaney's rectory window. He'd be reading a mystery novel under the lamplight near the coffee table. He'd get up and open the door and let in a parishioner who would sit in a high-back chair with news from the night: a death, a troubled child, an illness, a moved-out husband, missing money. Fr. Heaney would lean toward them, hovering like a statue, still, listening, the way he did in the confessional when his face was half hidden by the scrim of purple cloth. One time, Joey DePallo came in with a gun and handed it to Fr. Heaney. He knelt and Father made a sign of the cross on Joey's forehead — the way he did at baptism and confirmation — and picked up the phone. Two police cars arrived minutes later and Joey went away in handcuffs. A few church ladies would come in just to talk, leaving Bundt cakes and brownies on Father's desk. Nut and I never heard what anyone said. But you can know things without hearing, and in the narrow periphery of Nut's telescope you could see that language was more than words.

Another wave gathered. I rose toward the sky. I would have liked to have been alive when the pirates sailed this coast and the Indians hunted the rivers and marshes. Sphagnum moss holds eighty-one times its weight in water; we learned that in biology class. The quarterback for the Eagles practiced passing by throwing spirals through a tire swinging on a chain. Richard Nixon gave that silly over-the-head arm wave and disappeared in shame in a helicopter. He was a Quaker and his middle name was Milhous. Holy water and snowflakes felt the same on your forehead. I loved the scents of gasoline and chocolate, and of Mom's powder after her bath, but Mom was gone and even though Kurt kept her powder near the tub, the way he kept the Clabber Girl Baking Soda near the toaster, the same Clabber Girl that Mom had opened on the day she died, the scent was not the same. I liked Chick-O-Sticks, but not Jujubes; I didn't masturbate because I felt too alone afterward.

Kurt brushed alongside me.

"Let's swim in."

He beat me to shore. He rode a wave like a seal, skimming the foam of the white break, gliding to land and walking to dry sand where he plopped on his back, beads of water shining over his browning body. I caught a wave, but it slammed me hard, sucked me up, and slammed me again. I felt like a cartoon character in one of those inky, tumbling spirals. Mister Magoo. I dropped on the blanket next to Kurt.

"You want to lie on the blanket?"

"No," said Kurt. "The sand's heat feels good."

"Should we go check on Vera?"

"In a little while."

"I like this beach."

"Yeah."

"When are we going back to Philly?"

"Got to be soon, I guess. We're running out of money. It's amazing, Jim, how hard it is to put money in a wallet, but how easily it falls out. One day you're feeling rich with a bump in your back pocket, and then that bump gets smaller and smaller. What would it be like to be rich, really rich?"

"Like a rock star."

"Richer. My dad was always trying get-rich schemes. You know he painted ships like me, but he'd try to invent stuff on weekends. Once he invented a new car wax. He tested it on one of my Matchbox cars and it worked. Those little cars shined. But then he and I went out and rubbed it on the hood of our Buick and it left this dull, ugly smudge and my mom about killed him. I liked, though, that he kept trying to think of something new."

Kurt smiled.

"I wish we saw more of them."

"Maybe we'll go to Florida at Christmas. Dad likes to golf now. Seems to be what you do when you retire. Me, I'll play tennis. I'll live right next to a court in a warm place and play tennis every morning."

"Sounds rich."

"I'll never be rich, Jim. How about you? You gotta go to college. Your mom wanted that, and with all those words you know, it should be a cinch."

"I want to go, but I don't know what I want to be."

"Don't paint ships. The world is gray when you paint ships."

"Is that a joke?"

"I wish."

"Tell me about Mom."

The sun climbed higher. I heard a distant radio. The beach was filling up with wet dogs, Frisbees, coolers, and sandwiches wrapped in waxed paper.

"When we got married your mom told me she didn't want a big wedding. I said, 'Okay, let's have a small one.' I had just started at the shipyard, and I thought I'd invite a few friends and some family. But your mom said, 'Smaller.' What could be smaller? She said, 'You, me, and Father Heaney.' She didn't want a big show and a big white dress and flowers in the aisle. She said she just wanted to be there with me in the quiet of the church. She said all the other stuff would take away from what was happening between us. That's what we did. It was a Friday night in the candlelight of the church vestibule, your mom, me, Father Heaney, and an altar boy who slipped in at the last moment to hold the ring and be best man."

Kurt propped up on his elbows and looked to the waves.

"I loved that about her the most, Jim. Your mom loved strong but she loved quiet."

"Father Heaney must have been young."

"Younger and a little heavier, maybe."

"He's heard all my sins."

"What's he do with all of them: yours, mine, the whole parish? I wonder what it's like to match the sins of people with their faces."

"He can't see you through that purple cloth."

"He can see you just fine."

A Lab ran up and sniffed around me; its ocean-wet fur tickled.

"Why are we here, Kurt? With Vera?"

He bit his lip they way he did with Mom when he was stalling for time, not knowing exactly what to say.

"This woman, I can't explain, bringing in this energy and way to forget. I just want to forget, Jim, just for a little while longer what happened near that snowbank last winter, what we left in that graveyard. I know it can't be forgotten forever, but for a little while maybe we can get above it."

"But the gun and the man from Marrakesh."

"Think of her as Lizabeth Scott in tie-dye."

"That's not funny."

"I don't think there's a man from Marrakesh, Jim. There might be; I can't say for certain. That's the thing about Vera. I think her imagination has crowded in on her life. For most people, it's the other way around, but Vera is full of tiny worlds and many stories. I think, at least for now, she needs us and, Jim, we needed her."

"Do you love her?"

"No. But I'm learning there can be other things between a man and a woman. At first, I thought I was cheating on your mom. I'd think about that hard at night, but your mom, no matter where she is, knows my heart. We have to carry on, Jim, any way we can."

"Vera sure doesn't like Howard Johnson's."

"Probably why the relationship is doomed."

Kurt laughed. It was a strong laugh in the sun, near the water on the beach, mixing in with the wind and the waves like a part of nature. Do the dead look down from heaven? I decided not to ask Kurt. I lay back and thought about it myself, the sun warming my closed eyelids, making me see yellow-orange, a kind of glow, like being inside a broken egg. The man I met on the beach the other night, the science writer, he would have said no to my question. People can't peek from heaven because there is no heaven and there is no God; there are only bacteria and parasites, gnawing at the rims of good cells to sneak in and do damage. I was not that cynical, or maybe I was not that scientific. I believed in cells and spirits, a commingling of things like dead plankton floating, descending, falling onto the ocean bed or accumulating on reefs and the hulls of ships, giving new life, a kind of resurrection in the depths. Maybe it was that way in the sky and space, too, like those comets in Nut Johnson's telescope; they could be fiery, galactic matter as easily as they could be souls racing between purgatory and paradise.

Purgatory's a good word. It sounds and looks like what it is, a space, a floating wrinkle, or maybe a crack in the cosmos, a shelter or a holding cell, a place for sinners to purify before going to the light. Going to the light was a phrase repeated a lot by TV mystics — vacuum cleaner salesmen and women from New Mexico — who spoke of lying in hospital beds and glimpsing a tunnel and a light and feeling they should walk toward it. They never reached the light, never "crossed over" to the other side. They said it was God. I didn't trust them. An element of trust went missing when you appeared on talk shows like Mike Douglas or Merv Griffin. If there was a light, something out there beyond the knowing, I hoped Mom went toward it, that her spirit left her body and floated over that snowbank and up over our neighborhood and beyond Philadelphia, and that she found warmth and grace, not the kind the people talked about but the pure uncommercial kind, the kind you can't describe because the sensation is written with different words, words from another book, not the Bible, but a whole other book no one can decipher until soul and body part. I hoped that in the end the empirical (a word from biology class) and the spiritual became one.

I was sweating on the blanket; Kurt was sleeping in the sand. I sat up. The beach was full. I watched the girls in their bikinis; they moved like cheetahs. They were combed and polished, checking their tops and tan lines, flicking back their hair. The breeze from the shoreline snaked up the beach like the cool currents in the deep water where the waves gathered.

I saw Vera walking with her macramé purse and fedora straw hat. She wore a black bikini instead of her blue one-piece; her skin was pale and smooth, her black hair scattered over her shoulders, and in the distance she moved toward us in determined steps, her footprints deep and straight-lined in the sand as if she were following a map, not a circuitous map, but a map drawn by a hand intimate with the subtleties of the land. She spotted me watching her and waved. Her smile was big on her slim face, and I still couldn't tell if she was beautiful or not, but there was something about her that once you saw her you had to watch. I saw other men, their wives changing diapers or throwing Frisbees, watching, too. Maybe it was the color of her skin, or the way she moved, like a white stone melted to liquid. She looked like the Vera I had first met, not the one with the gun in her bag, but the one who on a rainy night in Philadelphia squeezed lemons into a pitcher and shoved it into our freezer. She was a little femme fatal, black and white and color, all at once; and maybe that was why the man from Marrakesh, if he existed, kept following her across America.

She sat in the sand. "I'm revived, Jim. I slept deeply and had many dreams, good dreams. I dreamed of a horse, a big white horse, a stallion, running through a souk and across the desert toward the sea. He had no rider. He was just big and free. His mane all tangled."

She glanced over at Kurt.

"Look at him snoozing. He looks like a big, sunburned child. We'd better wake him and turn him soon. Thanks for your note. When I woke up I looked from the balcony and saw you two on the beach, father and son. That's good, Jim. You think Kurt will like my new bathing suit?"

She got up and twirled. Her wet feet squeaked in the sand. I saw the raised circular scar, the color of cinnamon and milk, high on her leg. It looked like the first time I saw it: the circumference of a coin, a bullet hole, an indentation, a frozen ripple of gathered skin.

"I need a tan on my stomach, though. It's as white as new socks."

She sat beside me on the blanket and kissed my cheek.

"We're in no danger today, Jim. It's our day. Your day, my day, Kurt's day."

She leaned back, pulled her fedora tight, narrowing her vision. The sun was hot. I rose and went to the water, diving in without thinking about the chill, letting it jolt me, stinging my browning skin. I stood in the waves. They were gentler than in the morning. The tide was shifting around me, imperceptible, nature and the moon conspiring in their work, tugging at the great body of water, changing the lines in the sand. I looked to Vera, a faint shell dabbed with black. Kurt was still sleeping. Something pushed me. A splash. I went under.

"Boy, you better pay attention." Alice laughed as I surfaced. "I knocked you over easy."

She dove in and slid up my body, her skin as cool as shaved ice. She let go, twirled in the gentle surf, and dove in again.

"Why aren't you working? Who's at the front desk?"

"My uncle," she said. "I needed a swim and I saw you. How's your room?"

"Fine."

"Who's that woman with you and your dad? It's not your mom. I can tell a mom."

"She's a friend. Her name's Vera."

"She's strange. The other night, it was real late, maybe three AM, she came down to the desk. Gave me a startle. Her one hand was shaking and she was trying to hold it still. She asked if we had any city maps. I gave her one and she unfolded it. She said she needed a more detailed map with every street and road. I told her that's all we had. I smiled and said sorry. My daddy told me to do that when we couldn't meet the needs of our customers. I told her I'd try to get her a better map in the morning. She turned and went back to the elevator, not saying another word. It was strange, like she was sleep-walking or something, and the whole time that hand was shaking. Like it had a mind of its own."

"She's okay. She's just odd sometimes. She's traveled all over the world."

I wasn't going to tell Alice about Vera. We swam out to deeper water, our heads bobbing close to each other. Alice pulled up her top and hugged me while we floated. I had never felt a girl's breasts on me; it was blurry beneath the water and I couldn't see, but I could feel her shape pressed upon me; I could feel her cool, squeaky skin and the deeper warmth near her bones. Her body felt like two currents; her arms around my neck, I could hear her breathing in one ear, and I could hear the ocean in the other. I felt the world had shrunk, but I knew it hadn't, and all anyone on the beach could see, if they were looking at all, was our bobbing heads; everything beneath, her breasts, her knees, her toes dangling against my toes, was invisible, even to me.

The sun was moving away from us and over the land, and the moon was gathering in the sky, not too pronounced, but just enough to let you know that night was coming with the new tide. Alice was weightless in my arms, insubstantial, holding me, brushing against me as we floated. We seemed like two fish circling and touching each other. Slippery breaths. I kissed her, soft, like on the balcony the other night. She tasted of salt, of the sea, and she kissed back. The water held us. Cool and warm currents spiraled around, and Alice kissed me again, the water lifting us toward the moon. We dipped in the wake of a wave as it rolled toward shore and rose again on a new wave gathering below us. I opened my eyes. Alice's eyes were closed. Her hair floated on the water. We were far from shore, but I could see the umbrellas, like flowers in the sand, and the blankets, and the tall grass bending in the breeze on dunes near the houses with painted white window frames and cedar sides, some dark as mulch, others faded to bone. Alice stopped kissing me and slipped her arms from around me; she straightened her top and swam gracefully away. I followed with a breaststroke, my arms and legs out of rhythm, but I was moving forward, a vessel, trailing Alice to the shore. She rode a wave in as if she were born from water. I caught a slow wave farther out, riding in its middle, feeling it curl around me until it gently broke.

"I gotta git," she said. "I can't leave my uncle alone too long."

Alice stood; her top perfect, covering what moments ago had rubbed against me, elusive in the tide.

"I love it out there, don't you?" she said. "My daddy used to take my brother and me out in a boat, out farther then we were, and he'd make us dive in and swim to shore. He said, 'If you live on the water, you can't be scared of it.' It's the place I go when I want quiet and peace. Like a big watery church."

"I'm not such a good swimmer."

"You're a good floater." She laughed. "Like a piece of driftwood."

We stood looking at the waves. The air was cool.

"It must be nice here in a storm."

"That's the best time," she said. "The beach turns to gray, and the water is a pretty green, like a kind of precious stone, and the white of the waves is so bright they seem lit with electricity. It's like the ocean is cleansing itself. 'Angry and crashing.' That's what my daddy says. Which means it's time to nail up the plywood on the hotel window and drive inland to stay at my aunt's until it all blows out.

"How many more nights you staying?" she added. "The ledger says you're checking out day after tomorrow."

"I don't know. My dad hasn't told me."

"Maybe I'll come by later with some towels."

Alice winked. A shiny wink mixed with water and late sunlight. She kissed me on the forehead and walked up the beach, the wind lifting her wet hair, loose strands of it drying and making a haze around her like a gentle snowfall. I smiled, still thinking about her breasts. I didn't smile in the way that I had stolen something and gotten away with it; it was a smile, a feeling really, of being given something unexpectedly and not knowing if it would be given again. I imagined that's what loving a woman must be like, at least partly, waiting to be given things you most cherished, without asking and without knowing when they would be offered. I turned and looked. Kurt was sitting next to Vera, real close, elbows touching elbows. They both had their chins on their knees. I went to the boardwalk and ordered french fries from a guy in a shack with a window counter facing the ocean. I spoke through a screen; it was like sieving sins in a confessional. I couldn't see the man. I only heard his voice, saw his puffy hands, moving fast, flipping burgers, scooping pickle slices, spearing buns with toothpicks. I didn't know why he was working so fast. There was no line.

"Next," he said.

"There's no one else here."

"Did you order?"

"French fries."

"What time is it?"

"Late afternoon."

"And no one's behind you?"

"Nope."

"Huh."

He slid open the screen and stuck his head out, looked left and right.

"Huh," he said.

His face matched his hands, puffy, sweaty, and pinkish. He stepped out of the shack and came around from the side with my basket of french fries and a napkin. He wore a T-shirt, black-and-white-checkered pants, and an apron that once was white but had turned to a color I couldn't quite describe, maybe the color of cooling grease on a griddle, lardy, like schoolhouse paste. He was balding, but covered it with a comb-over of long black threads that curved around his forehead and whooshed back. Those threads looked miles long. His forearms were tattooed with mermaids.

"Catsup?"

"No thanks."

"I salted 'em pretty good. Buck twenty-five."

I pulled quarters from my damp pocket. The man studied the boardwalk.

"Maybe bad weather's coming, but it don't look like that. The sky's clear. Maybe there's a carnival. I hate 'em. Steal my business, bring in the riffraff. I'm usually busy this time of day. But it's all a mystery isn't it? Live here or vacation?"

"A trip."

"A trip? I suppose a trip is different than a vacation."

"Were you in the navy?"

"My girls give me away."

"My dad paints navy ships in Philly."

"I was in for twenty. Couldn't make chief and got out. Got these luvvies in the Philippines."

"You sailed all over the world?"

"Mostly the back side of it."

He checked his watch; studied the boardwalk some more.

"I can't figure this out. Been here five summers."

"A fluke. Unfathomable."

"Jesus, kid, cut it out. Eat your fries."

He smoked a cigarette in quiet.

"I'm going home. You want a hamburger? I made a dozen of 'em. It's on the house."

He went inside and slid a burger through the screen. I heard whistling and banging and pots clattering, the scrape of a spatula. He came back out with the apron in his hands and wearing a Hawaiian shirt with orange and blue flowers; the colors against the pants were alarming. He smelled of witch hazel.

"I'm off, kid. Clock-punched. Taking these ladies on the town." He lifted his arms. "Happiness on this one. Despair here. They look alike — twins, even —but they're different. See the faces?"

They were the same, except for their lips; curled up in one, curled down in the other.

"Isn't is amazing?" he said. "Just that slight difference changes everything. It's art. Like those masks of the ancient Greeks."

He walked away, apron string tailing behind, gulls flocking in the air around him.

That night I sat in Room 503. I waited for Alice to bring me towels. I watched the late news. High pressure hovered south and far away, no hurricane on the horizon, but possibly an eye was forming below Cuba. The weatherman would keep watch. I carved my name in a tiny bar of hotel soap; I turned the TV channels, sat on the bed, hummed "Helter Skelter," made muscles in the mirror, checked my tan face, so brown it made my teeth white as poured milk. I opened the dictionary to boredom and followed where it led. I threw the book aside; thought about Nut Johnson; thought about Kurt's forehand; thought about things that flashed in my mind for a second and disappeared, too brief to be cataloged; thought about Alice and cool, wet kisses in the sea, and it felt good to be expecting something, a knock on the door, a girl with towels, a Baptist with beautiful breasts I hadn't seen but had felt against me in the water's chill. I thought about the maps in Vera's purse; thought about votive candles in vestibules in winter, snow falling outside, cold, stained glass, purple, magenta, brightening amber; thought about the night, the black night beyond the waves, beyond the trawlers and freighters to continents in sunlight; thought about the world spinning, Galileo, the bones of saints, Black Sabbath, cartoons, *Leave It to Beaver* (what a dork); thought about Kurt hanging on a rope, the paint dripping in the water, coloring the fish; thought about tomorrow and how long it was going to take to get here.

A knock.

I swallowed, looked through the peephole. The bellboy uncle.

"Girl at the desk said you needed these."

He handed me two towels, turned, and walked down the hall, stutter-stepping, his shoulders slumped. The elevator opened. I heard a bit of the Beach Boys, then the elevator doors closed and the gimpy uncle descended to other tasks. I smiled. Girls were funny. I put the towels on the dresser and tiptoed to Room 501. I turned the doorknob and peeked in. Kurt and Vera were sleeping, a white sheet tangled between them. The hall light came through the crack in the door and shone on Vera's face. Her eyes opened, staring at me and then at the gun on the nightstand.

fourteen

"I don't suppose you remember the lemons of Sorrento, James."

"No."

"Bigger than a man's fist. They grow along the cliffs on the sea beneath Vesuvius."

"I don't recall seeing them, but I think Vera may have mentioned them once."

"The lemons there grow huge. Centuries of volcanic ash have made the soil strangely fertile. You loved them."

"I was there?"

"Yes, we ate salted meat and drank limoncello. Limoncello was your favorite. The taste is strong — can you remember the taste? The lemon scent fills your nose and the alcohol warms your tongue and seeps to your chest."

"Where are we?"

"The Jersey Shore."

"How long has it been dark?"

"It's just after sunset."

"The tide is moving."

"Like a carpet reeled out to sea. But you don't remember that, either?"

"No."

"A Turk told us that many years ago in Cyprus."

"I don't recall."

"We'll stay one more night?"

"Yes. I like it here. I like the ocean."

"We need more wine, James. We've drunk our Vranac."

A heavyset man wearing a ball cap and carrying two fishing poles and a tin bucket walks up the steps from the beach to the boardwalk. A woman follows, hauling two folding chairs. The man leans the poles on the railing and sets the bucket down. He squats and reaches into the bucket, pulling up a fish, a black ripple flapping in moonlight. It is fighting, but the tail fin wearies and the slap, slap grows fainter against the railing wood. The couple speaks, but I can't make out the words, only snatches of syllables when the wind shifts. They lay the fish on the railing and the man takes out a knife and guts it, the head falling into the sand, the belly slit. He cuts a piece and hands it to the woman, then one for himself. I smell garlic and other scents mixing in with the sand and salt. Gulls skim through the cone of boardwalk light, dipping toward the man and the woman, but then slicing into the black sky.

"I never could eat raw fish, James. But you like sushi."

"I smell garlic."

"Yes, and I think they're drinking vodka. They're speaking Russian. Can you hear?"

"What are they saying?"

"I'll whisper to you. I can't catch everything, but they're talking about fishing back home; it must be Russia, but I don't know where, and how much bigger the fish are, how much more they fight. The man says drink more vodka. The woman says she misses their son."

The woman kisses the man.

"He's in the army. Chechnya. The man says it's what the boy wanted, to stay in Russia and not move here with them. The woman says she wants to go back. It's not working here. The man says it takes time. The woman says there is never enough. The man says they'll get used to scrawny, timid fish."

The woman laughs. She puts her hand up to the man's cheek; her hand is white, fluttery in the moonlight. The man leans down and kisses her on the forehead. They sip vodka until the man grabs the bucket and poles and the couple walks away. The gulls descend on the railing, picking at the cut-open fish, flying away and eating bits of flesh atop the boardwalk lights.

"It's cold, James. Let's go."

The lady stands and takes my hand. My left foot is numb, but the tingle goes away as we walk. I don't know where we're going; I know this is the ocean and that the lady has a warm hand. I know my language. The lady tells me she is my wife. Eva. Have I heard this before? It seems I have, but I stop and look at her, a breeze blowing her dark hair across her face, the moon hardening, its light distinct. The lady is a white face aglow in the night. I look into her eyes and she puts a hand to my face and rubs my cheek as if I am an ancient lamp holding a genie. Why do I know about genies and not this woman? I can see in her eyes that she wants me to know. There's desperation in her eyes, not frantic, but worn.

"James?"

"Yes."

"I am Eva."

It's like a line from the Bible. Declarative, unadorned. But it registers nothing, except that she is here and, perhaps, I should believe her.

"I know only one part of my life," I say.

"I know of that summer, James. But your life is more, decades more. I don't want to talk about Kurt and Vera. There is so much more, James. You need to find it."

She takes her hand from my face. We turn and walk.

"I keep telling you stories. I am your memory. Your book. I have collected all of you so you're not forgotten. So *we're* not forgotten. There are two people involved; that's what the doctors don't understand. They're fascinated by you. How a young mind, a relatively young mind has become defective — they use the words defective and depleted as if you're a part in an engine or an isotope of uranium — twenty years earlier than it should be. Atrophies, thinning vessels, they describe your mind this way. They chart this. You are their experiment. I am just a lady at the edge of the couch. They bring me coffee and ask me questions, but it's only to humor me. They remind me of the bureaucrats in communist Poland."

"Poland?"

"Yes, James. My long-ago home."

"Where do you live now?"

"New York. In our apartment on the river."

"Do I live there?"

"No. You live somewhere else."

"A hospital?"

"A kind of hospital. Let me tell you another story. About us. We have so many stories, James."

The lady slows her step. She takes my hand again. We are alone on the boardwalk. There's a light in a diner, and past there, down an alley, a streetlight changes from red to green. Cars move, but not many; a man reads in a hotel lobby; the stained glass in a church glows in purple and deep red; a curtain in a home is drawn; nobody is on the boardwalk but the lady and me, walking in lights that seem bright puddles in the darkness. The lady's hand is warm.

"A story, a story, let me tell James a story."

She laughs. I am not a child.

"Don't be mad, James. I'm just kidding."

We stop at the edge of the light and lean on the boardwalk railing, the sea nearly invisible in the night.

"Budapest, James. A bar on the hill, just across the river from the Parliament. You know the one, like a pop-up in a story book. It was cold. A little snow that night as I remember. We had finished our interview. I think we were working on a story about what happened to old Soviet scientists. Those slippery creatures. We found a bar. It was hot inside. The windows were filled with steam and the place reeked of communist tobacco. Sweaters and coats strewn about and crowded with sweaty faces and arms, and then we heard it, the saxophone. Not playing Hungarian folk music, but jazz. Remember? You said, 'Who is that?' We pushed to the front. There was no stage, just a man with a saxophone playing near an upright piano.

"He wore a beret, a white T-shirt, and blue jeans. He was like wire. He held the saxophone slightly away from his chest; he bent forward as if he were bending a lover for a soft kiss in the middle of a slow dance. The music was scratchy, like raspy bubbles, each one distinct, long, floating through the bar like a pack-a-day smoker whispering secrets in the corner. That's what you said, James, and I laughed and laughed. You could be so full of yourself, so full of words. We stood with our beers and watched him. He never opened his eyes, remember? He just played, eyes closed and bent. You said he sounded like Ben Webster or maybe was it Coleman Hawkins. I didn't know. I just knew it was beautiful. I had heard jazz on smuggled records back in Poland, but had not seen the intimacy of it. It was erotic."

"Erotic?"

The lady smiles.

"What, you don't believe in the jazzman of Budapest?"

She fishes in her bag and steps under a boardwalk light.

"Read this headline: SAXOPHONE BLOWS BETWEEN TWO WORLDS.

"His name was Boris. He once played French horn in the Hungarian symphony. But jazz was the music he loved. He said he took tunes like 'Body and Soul' and turned them into his language, not changing them so much, but 'edging it' with his perspective, which he said wasn't that of a black American but of a Hungarian sick of the way most of his life had been lived behind a wall. He said he riffed misery. He played and drank until dawn, and then left the club to eat eggs and bread at a small café. He blew his sax softly over an espresso. He gave funny names to his songs: 'Apples and Apparatchiks,' 'Proletariat Moonlight.' He finished his breakfast and slipped his horn into a case, and walked out the door, a bent man disappearing in the morning fog. As he was leaving, he turned and said: 'Half a continent changing, believing in magic and Rice Krispies.'"

"What happened to the man?"

"I don't know, James. He told us he didn't know how to find 'the notes to this new life, this freedom.' That's what I always found so odd about your job, the journalist. You press so close to people. Get to know them in a compressed instant. You hear their stories, all unfolding like tiny plays. You write and take a piece of them with you, and then they are gone, fading further back in your notebook as new stories are told, listened to, collected. It's a strange intimacy you journalists have. I was the voice for all those stories, James. I was the translator."

"Did I write many stories?"

"Thousands."

"I can't remember a single one. How can I have written so many words and not remember?"

It is cruel to leave a man this way. The lady tells stories and I try to hold them, attach them to molecular structures, but memory is not there. I move my arm, wiggle my toe in a cold shoe, my brain works, but it can't summon memory, and all her sentences, I can't even remember how many she has spoken, they are like words written in white ink, shining for a moment before they disappear. I guess that's what's happening, but I can't say for sure. I can't say if I've been leaning on this boardwalk railing for days, years, or centuries. I like this woman. But I like her only in the instant; after that she's gone, and then another instant and that's gone. I want to believe her — but who knows how long this thought will last; it may already have disappeared. I touch her, I see her, I turn her face to the boardwalk light, nothing; only a pretty lady, like an ad in a magazine.

Turn the page, another face, another story, or are they the same face, the same story, page after page, denied recollection? I kick the boardwalk railing. I kick and I kick, and rage wells in me. I want to yell into the night, to scream my name and have my lost self echo back. I'm breathing hard and banging on the railing. I want to fight. I want to hit. I want to strike something to take the anger from me. But my arms get heavy and my breathing turns to weakened gasps, little misshapen puffs of fog in the cold night. I am a spent, useless storm. The lady steps back and then comes toward me, putting her hand to my cheek; it is a warm hand and she rubs my cheek as if she is polishing an ancient genie's lamp. Have I thought this before? Have I felt this sensation?

"James, it's okay. Calm down. A bad moment, just a bad passing moment."

She rubs my cheek. I feel her hand mix with water, smearing it in the cold night. I feel sweat on my back, my brow, but the rage is gone, curled back up, like my memory, in some hidden place.

"How long has it been night?"

"Two or three hours."

I am Jim. She calls me James. When did Jim become James? When did Jim get spots on the tops of his hands, gray hair on his forearms, wrinkles around his eyes, a crick in his neck? When did he age? What was it like? The body pulling ahead of the mind, leaving the mind behind, like a temple in a jungle. This thought disappears, too. Kurt, in that summer he told me to call him Kurt, one night pulled an abacus from his closet. It was old, with painted wooden beads. He'd had it since he was a kid. He said it was simple and exotic, that you could get to infinity by sliding beads. But I slide through the abyss. I am a broken abacus, beads skittering from side to side, numbers not adding up, infinity out there, or me lost in it. The lady kisses me on the cheek and wraps herself around me and I bend to hold her — I don't know why — and her mouth slides to my neck and warms me as the cold blows over my back and through my hair.

"Get a room."

The lady and I turn.

"Relax, just kidding. Nice evening. A little chilly, but you two seem cozy. Everything okay?"

"Yes, Officer," says the lady.

"Vacation?"

"Just out of the city for the weekend."

"That's good. Got to escape the grind every so often. Best time to be here, now and in the winter. It's almost here. I like the night shift in winter. Nobody on the beach. Nobody to cuff, no reports to fill out. None of the crazy shit the summer heat stirs up."

He steps to the boardwalk and looks over the empty sand to the sea.

"Sometimes, with a full moon, the surfers come. They're not supposed to, but I like watching them in the night. The cold doesn't bother those guys. Wet suits. They're mostly guys, but sometimes in the darkness you'll hear a girl's voice in the waves."

He has hair the color of a threatening sky and a full belly, a round man wearing a blue coat and a silver badge. His polished-brimmed hat rides high on his forehead and his face is meaty, pale, marbled with faint blooms of capillaries. Yet it's a nice face, inviting, coaxing. The radio on his shoulder coils up from his chest like a snake with a big head. His gun must be under his coat; he's bulky, rattling with metal and creaking with leather, breathing in the cold air, his green eyes watering, his gloved hands strumming the railing.

"It'll snow early this year."

He seems sure. He checks his watch. A big wave breaks.

"It's lovely, all this, don't you think?" says the cop. "The cold brings purity. I've always thought that."

The lady, the cop, and I stare at the ocean. His radio crackles.

"Charlie, we got a fire in a barrel out by the school. Probably just kids but you'd better check it out. Over. That Johnson kid. Over. Most likely. Over. On my way. Over."

The cop looks into the lady's eyes, glances at me and back to her.

"There's burning barrels and mischief in the night," he says, laughing and walking away, becoming one with the darkness.

The lady steps in front of me. "Let's dance, James."

She holds both my hands, and then slides one of her hands around my back. I put one arm around her. We stand like a wind vane. Still. I feel foolish. My feet are cold. No one is out. Just us in a circle of light, like a scene in one of those Lizabeth Scott movies Kurt liked so much. Lizabeth in a bedroom, long nightgown, a noise, eyes widen, the mouth tightens, a gun moves through the bedroom shadows toward the light. A scream. A pop. Music wells. Cut to a man in a fedora, smoking on a corner, looking to a window, seeing a silhouette . . .

The lady shuffles her feet, leans left, and guides me toward her. She shifts right and we do a little spin.

"There is no music, James. But there is the sea. Listen."

The sea is dull, a muffled roar trapped in a shell, distant, but rhythmic. I want to walk into the sea to drown this void, this not knowing. I know enough to know that I don't know. I am cognizant of my ignorance, that loss of self, except for that brief long-ago time (how long ago?) that I suppose now plays over and over; it's even playing now, dancing with this lady, who I don't know, but who says I do, who insists I do, but I do not. She whispers in my ear: Berlin, Prague, Budapest, Tirana, Trieste, Belgrade, Warsaw, Bucharest, détente, terrorists, Iraq, Iran, jihad, martyrs, suicide bombers, lemons, Sorrento, bandoliers, war crimes, mass graves, memorials, flames wisping from the earth, Montenegro, gunrunners, islands, sex, love, flowers, secret notes, a trip to Tunis, moonlight, pain, blood in a taxi, a baby lost, white linen, language, the meaning of words.

"Some things, James, are indescribable."

"Like what?"

"Hope."

We dance to the edge of the light. She stops, takes my hand. A dog runs out of the darkness, through the light, under the boardwalk railing and onto the beach. A young man follows in a sweater and a white scarf flowing like a ribbon. He nods and descends to the beach, running after the dog. The dog stops, bending down, leaning back, ready to spring. The man pulls a Frisbee from his sweater. It glows. Green. Like a spaceship, or a deep-sea creature. He throws it. The dog runs. Sand flies. The Frisbee soars, hovers, and is snatched from the black by the dog, who hangs briefly suspended over the waves; the sound of teeth clicking plastic. The dog runs to the man. The Frisbee spins again. The lady smiles. She rubs my cheek with a warm hand as if my face is an ancient genie lamp.

"One more night, James. Let's go to the hotel."

fifteen

Eva called again.

They drank wine, danced on the boardwalk, but nothing came back to James. Eva is upset. She is measured, but upset. She is learning that love has limits against the cruel designs of science and genetics. We spend most of our lives in between, I suppose, veering from one to the other until we are shriveled, put in the ground, or are burned and scattered in gray streaks across shorelines and valleys. My father, not my real father, but the man who adopted and raised me, Jeremiah, taught philosophy at a New Hampshire community college. His worldview was drawn from the philosopher Thomas Hobbes. Dinner table chat was brooding, recantations of misery pulled from that day's newspaper: starvation, coups, wars, plagues, and death. It was there, every day, the great Hobbesian creed played out with centrifugal force and written in the black ink of headlines. My mother, not Vera, but Connie, Jeremiah's wife, was a part-time nurse and social worker, and her inclinations were less foreboding than her husband's. Things, people, the planet and souls, yes, even winos, druggies, and murderers, could be redeemed. Saved.

"How can you wake up with no belief in the power of the human spirit to change things?" she'd say at the table.

"Tell that to villagers burned and singed, blistered by napalm."

I ate quickly when I was a child. One day I'd want to be a saint; the next a poet stewing in grim verse, like Rimbaud. I went into nursing. Maybe it was seeing Connie all those years in her folded white hat helping people in need. I don't know. I was good in science as a teenager, intimate with mechanisms, precise in biology, drawn to the frog in the jar and the clues beneath the scalpel's cut. I wanted structure and, not liking weapons or the prospect of barracks in distant lands, enrolled in nursing school and graduated a woman in white. I moved to Boston. My life was work, books, an occasional movie, an occasional party, brief affairs with surgeons and pharmacists; it's amazing how self-contained, how incestuous, the world of medicine is. My days were parsed into specific hours, my hand reaching through the dark to turn on a light to read until I could sleep again. Years went by.

I was working the night shift when Jeremiah and Connie, after returning from a party where everyone had to wear a T-shirt with their favorite Hobbesian quotation (Connie, the quiet, compassionate rebel, refused and chose a peace symbol), phoned and told me to come home for the weekend. They sounded nervous but assured me no one was ill; they said they had something they wanted to give me, something that should have been given years before. I couldn't imagine what it was, and, when Friday came, I left Boston in a flash, down the turnpike and through a dusk of autumn leaves. I opened the door to the Tudor house on Mill Lane and found Jeremiah and Connie sitting in the soft light beneath the kitchen table, where for so many years of my childhood we played Risk and Clue. They were holding hands. They turned and Jeremiah slid a worn envelope toward me. Connie was crying. I unfolded the letter.

"This tale, my daughter, is for you."

It took more than two hours to read. Jeremiah and Connie, who knew its contents, never moved. The only sounds were turning pages and wind at the back door. I finished the last page and folded my mother's words back into the envelope. I could feel tears on my face. I was born and taken from Vera and carried away. I was processed and fingerprinted, a picture of my infant face stapled to a folder. I was adopted and given a name. I was loved. Connie made tea and told me Vera died when I was six and that the letter arrived a year later through the adoption agency. There never was a right time to give it to me. Once when I was sixteen, and once when I was twenty-three, Jeremiah lifted it from its hiding place beneath the floorboards. But he never could put it into my hands. He didn't want the taint of an unknown ghost mother on our lives. That was selfish. I wanted to yell how selfish that was. I couldn't. I wasn't angry. I should have been, but nothing welled inside me, except the mystery of Vera and the revelation of James. I do not hold it against them, not too much anyway, the secret Jeremiah and Connie kept. I was their daughter before I could crawl. They bandaged, fed, and schooled me. They costumed me for Halloween, drove me to summer jobs, and held me through bad dreams. Could Vera have done more? But I remind them at least once a year now that if they had told me earlier, I could have found James before his mind crumbled. These words sting them but this is their penance. I am entitled to that. They are good people, they really are, dark and bright angels arguing over the world's ills, clinging to their love, a strange communion, like oil and water. I cherish them. But Vera's letter was vindication. There was something in me during childhood, not gnawing but ever-present, that suggested I was in the wrong place, like a picture tilted oddly on a wall. Where this feeling came from I do not know. We carry instincts into the world, woven into us before birth, intuitions there before learning. I never expressed this, never told Jeremiah and Connie of my faint estrangement to their love, but I felt the razor's edge of identity when I read Vera's letter.

What a letter it was, 133 pages; some written in longhand, some typed; some pages flowing with ornate penmanship, others a jumbled, dizzying thicket of words. I read of Egypt, deserts, souks, the Red Sea, the Dead Sea, horses and tents, ablutions, drinking wine and making love in whitewashed bungalows with sea-blue shutters. It wasn't a letter. It was an autobiography of a mother. My mother. The man from Marrakesh was there, a lover at first, but growing more sinister as Vera's story unfolded and her alphabet turned blockish with demons, yes, tiny devils drawn and lurking between q's, g's, and o's.

Page 107: "He was there today, but I couldn't see him, although I spotted him yesterday, slipping around the corner behind me, like a breath, a wicked breath. He will kill me. But when? I am an antelope; he a lion. The watering hole is shrinking. No one believes me. That's because he's clever, clever like the night. He will find me here, even in this place where the white shoes squeak and the windows are crisscrossed with wire. My daughter, wherever you are, believe what others do not. He is here. Omnipresent. Dust gathering and dispersing in an ancient wind. How old are you, my daughter? I do not know. They've taken my calendars, my maps. They even took you. You never suckled from me. They laid you blue and bloody on my belly, my legs splayed, held apart by shiny metal. I felt your life, your heat. You seeped into me. And then they carried you away, out a swinging door. Down the hall. Squeaking. If I can escape here I will find you. I will draw new maps and find you . . ."

It is not coincidence that I am a nurse and James is a man in need of a nurse. The world has joined what should have been bonded all along. The hand of God reaching through His sea of mortals has set something right, or maybe it's just the power of nature to reunite blood. I am the woman in white. I stand guard over my half brother. He is fading, I know. He doesn't know me. I haven't told him yet. I haven't told Eva, either. James doesn't know that his skin, his pigment, the color of his eyes, the way he dips his head to the left when he listens are all me, too. I wonder sometimes that others don't see the obvious.

In the morning, when I go into his room and open the curtains, I wonder if this will be the day that the sunlight hits him just right and brightens what's dark in him. I know better. I am a nurse; I know biology, the sciences of decay. I chart with precision. But we can hope. People wake from years-long comas; drowning men are pulled from the sea.

Vera's letter. Page 121: "My daughter. What have they named you? There is something you must know. Something to make you complete. You have a brother. I guess he is a half brother, since you are my only child. His name is Jim. He is thin the way boys are thin, unformed, knees, elbows, and arms, but you can see where the muscles and lines will be. Boys are like that, growing from the inside out. His mother died. But his father is your father. Jim reads the dictionary. All the time. He slips big words in, so you have to watch. A conversation is going along and then, out of nowhere, a strange word warbles out of his mouth. It's cute. Jim is cute. I've lost him. I've written him letters, but have heard nothing. His last name is Ryan. He's from Philadelphia. I don't know if he ever believed me about the man from Marrakesh. Things ended quickly with us. I don't know when, or if, you'll ever get this letter. I'm looking at all the pages now; it's certainly grown into a very, very long letter. A confession? An apology? I keep it in a folder. The people here are nice that way. Time, as I mentioned earlier, is vague to me. I can't seem to grasp a minute, and I don't know if the minutes are flying past, or dripping by, one slow drop at a time. But Jim will be out there. He may be a lot older, become someone much different than who I remember. But I remember him well. His hair going every which way in that Impala. His face tan. His diving into waves and laughing, and the way he looked at me sometimes, like I was a bird flown in from a distant wind. Sometimes he would smile and look down, bashful, as if he couldn't figure me out, even with all his vocabulary. He liked the Beatles. The *White Album,* if I remember correctly, was his favorite. That is Jim.

"And now I have to tell you about your father. His name was Kurt. He painted ships and played tennis. It was in the morning I lost him. I think just before dawn; the air had that speckled, fuzzy grayness. It is a conspiring time when night meets the coming day. Things appear not as they are. Nothing is certain in twilight. You will learn this. Kurt was in the twilight, but there was another shadow commingling, too. You know, if you've read this letter, who that shadow was. He was there. I know it. He was moving behind Kurt, slinking like he did, like he did so many times, like a spirit, a jinn, but this time he was so much closer, there in the twilight with Kurt and me. Kurt didn't see him, because as I told you, he was behind Kurt. I reached into my bag. It was a big macramé purse. I felt the handle. The next thing I knew, light had filled the room. Men with dark suits and radios surrounded me. They kept asking me questions. Writing things with their little pencils . . ."

Vera's eyes locked on mine. The crack of the door sent a blindfold of light across her face, like in those horror movies when the girl, usually a virgin or a babysitter, hears a sound downstairs in a big house on a windy night. The camera moves with the stealth of a spider, capturing the girl's darting, spooked eyes, black doll's eyes, while a tree branch scratches at the window and dead leaves blow in a courtyard. Vera looked to the gun on the nightstand, reached for it, but then must have recognized me. Her hand retracted under the white sheet and she curled around Kurt, who was in a deep sleep, his head tilted toward the open curtains to the balcony and the sea.

"Go to bed, Jim," came Vera's voice from the darkness.

I closed the door to Room 501 and tiptoed back to 503. I sensed somebody in the hall, just around the corner, but I heard no key slide and figured it was Alice's gimpy uncle walking his night rounds, counting bars of soap and bottles of shampoo, inspecting shower curtains in vacant rooms, fixing the housekeeper's cart, ordering more toilet paper, tinkering with the hidden machinery of the hospitality industry. I went inside and closed the door. Turning on the TV; turning it off. Flicking through the Bible and looking under the bed to see if an earlier guest had left something of value, some clue to bring two strangers together. A hotel room is a prison cell when you can't sleep. The breeze billowed the muslin curtains; they seemed like big white lungs in the darkness, filling and collapsing, breathing. I went to the balcony.

"Out wandering, boy?"

Alice sat staring at the ocean through the railing.

"What are you doing?"

"Counting waves. Four hundred and seventy-three. Shouldn't leave your door open. Don't know who could come and gitcha in the night. My daddy says at hotel conventions managers tell stories of all the strange, unexplainable things that happen in their hotels. My daddy figures hundreds of people a year disappear from hotel rooms. Just vanish, like they were kidnapped by space aliens."

She turned toward me, an ember like a firefly lighting her face.

"You wanna hit?"

"You Baptist girls sure smoke a lot of dope."

"Tonight's my night off."

"Who's at the front desk? Your uncle?"

"No. This guy Slim. Daddy knows him from church. He was gonna be a preacher but didn't have the calling."

"The calling?"

"The gift."

She sucked again; the glow around her face brightened.

"The gift is speaking the words as if they were written just for you. Some preachers have it, most don't. My daddy calls it 'magnetism.' He says only God can put it on your tongue."

She switched the joint to her other hand, blew its ash into the night, and relit it with a silver lighter.

"Wasn't the ocean nice today? I liked being out in there with you," she said. "I liked kissing and floating, the currents spinning us slow."

"I never kissed in the ocean before . . ."

"Bet you never saw a girl's breasts in the ocean before, either."

She laughed. I blushed, but it was night and Alice couldn't see. I took the joint.

"I didn't really see them. The water obscured the detail."

"I could take that as an insult if I knew what obscured meant. You ever think how you'll die?"

"No."

"I do sometimes. I think it's church. Preachers make you feel like there's so much out there. Like the world is full of tiny, invisible traps of darkness. If I could choose how I'd die, I'd choose the ocean. Being swept out gently by the currents, the water turning colder and colder and my body going numb, slowly filling, all the time having the sensation of floating, like a sea angel flying on the tide toward God."

Her voice was a little cracked from the smoke; it was huskier, but soothing. I closed my eyes and listened. She was a radio in the night, talking into the ether, making shapes with sounds in the scratchy distance. I wasn't high. I was simply peaceful. Vera's hand was off the trigger and all seemed quiet in 501, while in 503 a girl with breasts, a lighter, and a bag of her brother's marijuana talked and talked, a merry-go-round of words, raspy against the waves. I heard a crinkle.

"You want half? Milky Way. I got it from the box we stock the vending machines with."

"You must have a lot of stuff like that, supplies I mean."

"A truck is always dropping something off. One time we had three deliveries of soap in one day. It was a screwup, but we had all this soap and Daddy said it was enough to wash every soldier in the entire US Army. It was in winter and there were hardly any guests, so you know what we did? We lined the soap up like dominoes, setting them up in the shape of a Tilt-A-Whirl, you know, a spiral tightening. And then we let 'em fall. It was beautiful. They fell so fast and they made a kind of soft clattery music."

"Do you like the Beatles?"

"Didn't they break up?"

"Yeah."

"I'm still hungry. I got another candy bar. Want half?"

"Sure."

"Almond Joy. Shit. I meant to get Mounds. You can have my almond."

Alice flicked the joint over the railing. We ate in silence, Alice handing me her almond. When she was done, she stepped over to where I was leaning and kissed me. We tasted almost the same. She kissed me the way she did in the water. Soft. I felt her back, bare in her halter top, and it was warm, as if her skin had stored up the day's sun. Her hair smelled of dope and the sea, a little perfume on her neck. She pressed against me and lifted a hand to my cheek and then another, holding my face as if it were something delicate, like crystal or the blown glass of a Christmas ornament.

She kissed me again. Brief. Her tongue traced my chocolate lips and I felt that somehow she was older, older in the way that girls are in elementary school, when they are better than the boys in penmanship and arithmetic. Maybe she was a little scared like I was, but I didn't think so, she seemed to know about skin and kisses, and how to blow a breath across a neck. She took my hand and led me through the curtains into the dark room and onto the bed. We lay like fallen wood, side by side, pressed together, but then, like we did in the ocean, we seemed to float. I opened my eyes and in the bits of gray and dark I saw her looking at me, not like Vera with her gun, not scared and waiting, but looking at me like I was her own private mystery, a boy on a bed in her daddy's hotel, floating with her above the waves in the warm stillness of her breathing. I stroked her hair.

"You still checking out day after tomorrow? Your daddy and that woman he's with haven't changed the reservation."

"I don't know what we're doing."

She kissed me again, then sat up and took off her halter top. She lifted off my shirt, and we lay back down. I didn't know what to do; boys pretend but they don't know, and I didn't know. She took my hand and put it on her breast. Nothing was blurry like it had been in the ocean. Even though it was gray-dark, her breasts were white, blooms of white, a girl's unfinished white, rising from her tanned body.

"Can you feel my heart?"

"It's going fast."

"I feel it, too. We can't do no more than this, Jim. Just this kissing and touching."

"That's okay."

"You taste like a big candy bar."

She laughed and rolled on top of me, her hair fell around me, and she lifted and dipped, like a kite, on my breathing. I didn't know what to say. I said nothing. I was glad we weren't going further, to a place I didn't know. Part of me wanted to, but most of me didn't. I wasn't an altar boy. I wasn't gay, but I wasn't a Beatles' *White Album* song, either. Alice made me feel like a boy sensing his manhood out there a dozen waves from shore, gathering but not yet arrived. Her voice made me imagine I was kissing Lizabeth Scott. The tone vulnerable, a voice of hurt or waiting to be hurt; Alice's voice invited you in, wrapped you up like you were her conspirator, but then it held you at bay. She sat up and straddled me.

"Trace me."

"What?"

"Trace me with your fingers. Trace me and you'll never forget me."

I traced her. It seemed I was cutting her from the night. Neck, shoulders, down the arms, elbows, hands; skimming her waist, up her stomach to her breasts and around them, moving to her collarbone and slipping over her chin, like slipping over a dune, to her face, her forehead, my fingers disappearing into her hair. I did it twice. She lay beside me, the way Mom used to lie beside Kurt on the couch after a long day.

"Let's sleep," said Alice. "When you wake I'll be gone, and you'll wonder if this all ever happened."

"I traced you. I'll remember."

I closed my eyes. I could feel Alice's heart beating beside mine. I wondered what we would look like in Nut Johnson's telescope. Two specks of flesh in the night — a boy and a girl — tangled together by kisses and arms, and sleeping in a room by the sea below the great constellations and the ghosts of old sailors who charted the stars toward doom or fortune. I could talk to Nut like that. He would understand. He would see me through his telescope and know that something had happened, that I was the same, but somehow changed; that seeing a girl's breasts, touching them, having them press against you was wonderful, but not in the way a boy expects in his mind before it actually happens. It's different. Better. But somehow you feel tricked in the nicest kind of way. Nut would know this without my having to explain, just like he knew, when peering at Mrs. Romano's silhouette through her lighted shade, the splendor of shadows that spin before us.

The morning light glared harsh. I turned and squinted. Alice was gone. She left me the nub of a joint in the ashtray and an Almond Joy wrapper on the TV. She had been here. It was real. I closed my eyes and retraced her once more in my mind. I wanted it etched deeply. A knock and the door flew open.

"There are strange goings-on, Jim. I need to play tennis. Let's go."

"I'm a little rusty."

"You'll be fine today."

Kurt handed me a Jack Kramer racquet, a towel, and a can of balls.

"Where's Vera?"

"We'll talk about Vera later. We need to find a court."

Down the elevator to the lobby; Slim, a raggedly thin, aptly named man, a man without the preacher's gift, without God's blessings on his tongue, sat where Alice usually sat, looking over the ledger at the front desk while the gimpy uncle sipped coffee. Slim gave us directions to a high school with good courts about five miles away.

"Have a wonderful game, gentlemen," he said.

Kurt and I dropped the top on the Impala and took off with a roar through sparse Sunday-morning traffic. Kurt popped in Walter Jackson and that big, deep voice filled the air like its own kind of church. The sun was warm, but the breeze was cool, and as we drove the ocean's stickiness thinned. Nobody was on the courts. They were smooth with evaporating dew, the white lines bold, the green uncracked, like a gardener's lawn on the Philly Main Line. Kurt opened a can, a snap and a whoosh of air and the gluey locked-up smell of new balls.

"Swing easy like I taught you."

"That was a long time ago."

"Just easy long strokes, don't hurry, just glide to the ball."

I hadn't played tennis with Kurt in two years. He hit softly so I could find a rhythm. It took a while. I sent balls streaming over the fence and skidding across other courts. Kurt kept saying: "Relax . . . Long strokes . . . Get your racquet back . . . You're hitting too late . . . You're hitting too early . . . Topspin . . . Roll the wrist . . . Relax." One good thing about Kurt — he seldom got mad, rarely raised his voice. Tennis was his passion, and he did not like to see it played poorly, but he was patient, knowing that this game of mathematics and art needed time and humor; otherwise a man would throw tantrums and smash a lot of Jack Kramers.

This was the Kurt I knew from Philly. The Kurt of Mom and me. Lately, with his uncombed hair and tan, and his unconcern for detail, like having a clean white T-shirt or stiff, newly washed jeans, Kurt, who even let slip his meticulous care of the Impala, a sandy rolling box of crumbs and soda stains, was a different shade of himself. Vera had done it, which when it first happened was good, watching Kurt, like a snail peeking out after a rainstorm, come back to the light after Mom's death. She drew me out, too. She enchanted.

Kurt was out too far, though. He wanted the cover of his shell again, he wanted to paint ships gray and hang from rope ladders. I didn't ask him about this. I saw it. Vera, the one who drew him into the light, was losing herself, reaching for a gun and scrunching up scared in the night; she could no longer keep Kurt in her fairy tale. That sounds strange, but I think it was a fairy tale. I wanted there to be a man from Marrakesh clawing outside the fortress walls, not for the danger or a boy's adventure, but so Kurt and I could have faith.

Faith was a never-ending work in progress. I wished I had more of it, but I often felt faith was a trick on the spirit. Was Christ really on your tongue at communion? Did His body and blood dissolve into yours and flow through your veins to make the impure holy? Faith and mystery were twins. That's what Fr. Heaney preached; that's what made a tiny moon of unleavened bread the body of God's son. You could doubt that, even as you knelt while Fr. Heaney rummaged his stubby fingers in the gold chalice and plucked up your Christ and held Him before you as you uttered "Amen" and crossed yourself and walked to your pew with the Lord sliding down your throat and into your soul. Kurt believed in God and communion but the tennis court was what he most trusted, the place that no matter where he went was the same divine rectangle of familiarity protected by a fence that held back parking lots, tall grass, and other annoyances seen and imagined. I watched him on the other side. He was beautiful when he moved. His body born for the game; bone and reflex synchronized to the swoop of his racquet, an arc of symmetrical perfection as precise as the twitch of a swan's wing. The ball lifting off the strings and finding the invisible weight of topspin as it accelerated and dipped over the net like a piece of light. He kept me running, side to side, up to the net, back-footing it to the base-line. I wasn't beautiful. I breathed hard and played with abandon, and I could hear Kurt laugh across the net, not making fun of me but admiring, maybe it was admiring, the strange, gangly theater of my game.

"You've got your own style," he said walking to the net to pick up balls.

"Looks funny."

"No, Jim, it doesn't. It's unique and there's nothing wrong with that. A man needs uniqueness in his life. It sets him apart, you know. Nothing wrong with that. Keep being unique, Jim. The world has a way of wanting to take that away from you."

"You feel unique?"

"In moments."

"Vera's unique."

"That's one word for it."

"This girl Alice at the front desk, she's unique."

"What's going on with her? I saw you two swimming beyond the waves the other day."

"We're just friends."

"Women are unique by nature."

"Maybe."

He slipped a ball into his pocket and looked at the late-morning sun. Sweat shone on his face and beaded at the tips of his long hair. His white shirt was drenched. It was a moment he wanted to keep in a bottle and twist shut. You can tell when a man feels that way; there's a smile, but not a full one, the shoulders slump a bit, and the legs seem balanced on oiled springs; a man is quiet at this moment; feeling like the speck he is in the world is brightened, made known. To speak would wipe it away; to make a sound would be to lose the true, unpronounceable thing that gives him the measure of who he is. I wasn't a man, but I studied men. I studied Kurt, and while a lot of him had changed since we met Vera, his pose of contentment, like the way he sipped a beer on the summer stoop or how he used to look at Mom when she pulled something sweet from the oven, had not changed, although it had become harder to find.

"Alice wears mostly halter tops, doesn't she, Jim?"

"A different color every day."

"Like pulling flags from a drawer."

"She's a Baptist."

"Not many of them in Philly. Nuns and girls in plaid pleated skirts. When I'm late for work and stuck in traffic, I see all those Catholic girls, holding books to their chests and hurrying in packs to school. When I see them it's like being young and being old at the same time."

"You're not old."

"Some of those girls will marry men like me and move into row houses and raise families. Others will move to Rittenhouse Square and be secretaries and accountants. A few will leave and won't come back."

Kurt took the ball from his pocket and bounced it on his racquet as he spoke. He didn't look at it; he just kept it bouncing like a thing with its own life.

"Your mom and I knew a girl who left. She was from St. Thomas's and she was a genius. Her father was a cripple and her mother had run off. The girl raised herself and cared for her broken old man. He drank too much but he was a gentle drunk. I was in her house a few times. It smelled like Pledge. Her name was Mary and man, could she do math. Whole pages of numbers and graphs and squiggles I couldn't even begin to understand. She was communicating with a whole other world. The nuns didn't know what to do. They couldn't keep up with her. They brought in college professors. I felt sorry for her. She was this quiet thing no one could figure out. Our neighborhood mystery. It was the first time in my life that I really understood how different people are. You grow up in a tight neighborhood of alleys and brick homes and everyone knows everyone from the shipyards and the factories, everyone's connected and you feel that they're all like you. But they're not. The ones like Mary let you know that. I asked a nun about Mary and she said, 'God dispenses His gifts in different quantities.' I'll never forget that."

Kurt's voice was low and soft.

"Mary disappeared after graduation. She went to schools in New England and sometimes her dad would mix her into his drunken stories. 'Mary was working on something for the government.' 'Mary was splitting atoms.' Mary never came home. Not for Christmas. Not for anything. Not even for her father's funeral. One day I was reading the *Inquirer* and saw a headline: BRILLIANT PHILLY-BORN SCIENTIST DROWNS. There was a picture of Mary. She had kept those same pointy-framed glasses and that funny sideways part in her hair. But she was gone, leaving behind, the paper said, a three-room apartment and unfinished theories. She drowned in Walden Pond outside Boston. Fell through thawing winter ice. I thought, How could that be? How could a girl so smart not know the dangers of thawing ice? All that math and all those numbers in her head. She must have felt the temperature. She must have seen the sheen of water on top of the ice. But she fell through. The smartest person I ever knew drowned like a child or a fool not paying attention."

"Maybe it was suicide."

"There was no note. No inkling of it. Her scientist friends said she was excited, that she was about to solve an unsolvable equation, or some scientific thing."

"Maybe in the end she couldn't solve it."

"No, Jim. It didn't feel that way. You don't kill yourself in a half-frozen pond. Mary was too smart. She would have thought of a better way. But if she was that smart, why did she fall through? I keep thinking about that. It's strange. The way your mom died is not strange to me. A car slides on the snow, jumps a sidewalk, and hits someone. That's freakish, but I can see it in my mind. The puzzle of it solved. Witnesses said the car went out of control in bad weather. But Mary through the ice I can't get."

"But Mom's puzzle is not solved. We never found out who was driving that car. No one ever got a license plate number, or they were too scared to come forward with it."

"You know who was driving that car."

"A numbers collector for the mob."

"That's the kind of car it was. A black Fleetwood."

"How do we live with that, Kurt?"

"We put it away. Store it deep somewhere. I figure it like this. Whoever hit her, hit her by accident. The crime was in driving away. That's what I hold to, Jim. It gets me through. But one day, and you know how Philly is, I'll be working at the shipyards and someone'll whisper into my ear the name of the man who was driving that car. Then, I think, real quiet I'll go see that man one night. You can't act on anger. You got to let things settle. Let them harden so you can see clearly. Waiting can kill a man, but waiting, my dad used to call it 'biding time,' is what you have to do sometimes."

"I want to come when you go see that man."

"Maybe. Keep one of your dictionary pages open to patience."

Kurt was still bouncing the ball on his racquet, but the racquet had switched hands.

"Nimble."

"What?"

"You're nimble. That's my word for you today."

"Procrastinator. As in a boy delaying getting his ass kicked in tennis by his old man. Get back over there and let's hit."

I smiled and ran to the baseline, my legs stiff from standing so long at the net. Kurt's balls came quick, precise, smudging the white lines, every one in but every one so close to being out. Kurt said the key to the game was taking space away from the opponent, gradually shrinking where the opponent could go, and then, just at the right moment, putting the opponent on the run. He said "opponent" when he played tennis. He didn't say *guy* or *man*. I was his opponent on the court, not his son. I was somebody to be beaten. I liked that. I liked that he thought enough of me to give me his best. That's what a boy wants most from his father. The respect of being counted as an equal, of losing, maybe, but keeping that respect until the day he wins, which I was sure must feel like it felt when I traced Alice in the darkness.

Kurt beat me 6–0. We played a second set and I lost 6–0 again, but I hit better and found angles that surprised Kurt a few times. I even slid an ace by him. An old couple played on the court next to us. Their skin was the color of pancake batter; webs of purplish veins ran through their legs. They wore long visors and big black sunglasses. They seemed uncommonly pale. I had to squint to look at them. They were consistent but what little power they had was all above the waist. Theirs was a languid game, the ball a burned-out planet, arching and landing with no spin, but staying in play as if you took the game that was in them long ago and set it to slow motion. Kurt and I studied them from the fence shade.

"The legs go first on an athlete," said Kurt. "Look at the guy. He shuffles and his swing is stiff. What's that word, Jim? He's lost his, ah . . . fluidity. That's it. He's lost his fluidity. He's doing okay for an old guy, but you hate to see it happen, don't you? I bet he can remember those days when his legs worked just fine. I bet he can see his game like his memory sees it."

"It's good that they're hitting at their age, though."

"No doubt. That's how I'll be one day. An old man with a can of balls, roaming tennis courts looking for games. Everything slower. Knees stiff. Ankles brittle. Shoulders cramped. Aging is like going into battle day after day. That's what it seems like to me. Just so long as I keep my mind, remember what I know now about chasing balls and hitting angles. If I keep up my leg squats maybe it'll be a long time before I slow down. It's all about strong muscles."

Kurt built his muscles in the basement of our Philly home. Like the back stoop he sipped his beer on after work, the basement, an unfinished, unpainted cave at the bottom of twelve narrow steps, was his place, except for the washer and dryer Mom had under a lint-shrouded window that let in strangled strands of light. When I went down, which wasn't often, to hunt for a shirt or a pair of socks in a pile of laundry, it was an underworld of brass and copper pipes, slanted beams, half-driven nails, wires, circuit breakers, and gray metal boxes, the bones and veins of a house, absorbing and bending with footsteps that creaked like ghosts just beyond the square of light in the kitchen above.

Kurt kept his weights and barbells on a ripped rug near the drain in the center of the cement floor. A punching bag, suspended on silver chains, hung near the water heater whose blue flame glowed in the corner and seemed, to a kid's imagination, an uncharted galaxy. Kurt had wanted to be a boxer when he graduated high school. He was a Golden Gloves prospect and the guys in the neighborhood and a few lines in the *Inquirer* had summed him up not as a natural but "a tough brawler who could take a punch." Philly didn't care much about prettiness; it was a city of looping fists and spat blood, a black-eyed and bruised small-town metropolis, much different from New York to the north, which seemed to me, on my one visit there on a field trip to the Museum of Natural History, to be splendor built on artifice (one of my first dictionary words). Being labeled "tough" in Philly was like having a seat at the Round Table.

One night after hurrying to a bout through a rainstorm, Kurt broke his right hand on the jaw of a counterpuncher from Asbury Park in round three of his tenth fight. He wore a cast for a month, which meant he couldn't play tennis, a love he had kept a secret from the guys at the Kensington gym. Not having a racquet in his hand for so long seemed unnatural to Kurt. He quit boxing. He wasn't going to be a great fighter; he'd have been a pugilist who'd have hustled with his gloves, rubbing alcohol, shoes, and workout bag from Atlantic City to Hoboken but never to the Spectrum or the Garden. Kurt saw through his dream early, saw in his mind, I suppose, what his body and luck could not achieve, not like a lot of Philly guys with crooked noses and scars under their eyes and stories of winter nights and icy rings in armories scattered through the Pinelands.

Kurt wasn't ever going to touch the grass in Wimbledon, either, but tennis was the image of himself he wanted. It was what he trusted. Every autumn, when the rains came and the court nets were dropped and folded away, Kurt would tape his knuckles and hit the punching bag, light jabs at first and then, as the sweat came, harder body shots, making the bag shimmy and jump on its chains so it seemed Kurt and the bag were dancing in our basement. The kitchen floor shook, the living room floor shook. It could happen at any time. Kurt kept no set workout schedule, and sometimes Mom and I would be awakened at three or four in the morning by the slap-sound of the bag and the grunts and the rolling-metal clatter of barbells and weights dropping and gyrating on the basement floor like big nickels warbling on a countertop.

One time, maybe about three months before Mom died, I snuck downstairs in the hours before dawn and saw Kurt leaning back on a kitchen chair drinking a beer, knuckle tape dangling in strands, sweat pouring off him; he sat there until first light came through the window over the sink. It is the most amazing time when dawn strikes night. Kurt stood up that morning and scrambled eggs in a black skillet, whistling, his back slick. He didn't see me. I slinked back upstairs and a few minutes later, I heard Kurt (he was Dad back then) open his bedroom door and I heard covers rustle and Mom laugh and the door shut, not with a slam but with the hushed click of a secret.

I eased back on the fence and watched the old couple. They leaned their racquets on the net and shared a water bottle from a cooler. They talked and pointed, reliving strokes and rallies the way you might reminisce over scrapbook pictures. I nudged Kurt. He rolled his eyes. I nudged him again and pulled up my sleeve and flexed.

"I've been working on my muscles, too."

Kurt cracked up.

"Jesus, Jim, you're gonna hurt yourself. Where is that little bump hiding anyway?"

I cracked up, too.

"You can use my weights when we get back to Philly."

"When are we going?"

Kurt rested his head on the fence and closed his eyes. His smile died. He was silent for a while before he spoke.

"I'm worried about Vera. She's not right. She can still be magical in that way she is. But she's losing her grasp."

"The other night I peeked into your room and she was staring at the gun on the nightstand."

"She's convinced that man is out there. But there's no man. If there was, if he is like she says, he would have come long ago. We just can't leave her. We've got to get her help. I feel bad about it. But I don't regret taking this trip. As a father it maybe was not the best idea, but I never felt in danger, even from the beginning. I just figured we were living out one of Vera's stories. I can't explain it. She's so different from me, but I think I wanted to hide in Vera's stories. All those places out there she brought to us."

"Do you think she was ever in the deserts and the Maghreb?"

"I don't know, but they sound pretty."

"It's hard to tell what's real and not anymore."

"What do you think?"

"Sometimes I think I see a shadow or feel a presence, as if someone is there watching us. When I turn there's nothing."

"The mind plays tricks. She's got us half believing . . ."

We packed our racquets and walked past the old couple who had returned to the patter of their strokes. Kurt took off his wet shirt and grabbed a dry one from the Impala's trunk, which had started to look like the closet of a traveling salesman: tools, jack, and spare tire covered in a jumbled tide of clothes, cups, blankets, paper bags, magazines, Vera's underwear, straw hats, and the stuff that accumulates on a trip with no specific destination. The top was down and the sun seeped into the leather seats, and even though I was hot from playing tennis, the warmth of the car felt good. I leaned back and closed my eyes. Kurt slipped us into traffic and after a few minutes, amid a scratchy Walter Jackson ballad and the rattle of Sunday churchgoers, I smelled the sea air and thought of what it would be like to gallop on a horse across a North African beach, splashing in the surf beneath cliffs and racing through whitewashed villages with blue and green shutters, and into the great souk, dipping my hands into sacks of cumin and saffron, and sitting in a café sipping tea, an overhead fan stirring the musty, ancient air around me. What's wrong to think like that? To be in a place so strange? Maybe Vera wasn't there, or maybe she was. How can you tell stories so precise if they are not real? How can you conjure worlds so intimate if they're false? Threads of gasoline coiled through the sea breeze. I heard snatches of passing radios and felt the Impala turn a corner. The air turned hot, sugary, and butter-smeared. I opened my eyes. Kurt parked in front of a Krispy Kreme.

"I've heard these are the best donuts. They don't make 'em up north."

Kurt went in and I could see him through the big spotless window, standing in line at the counter, among people sitting in red swivel seats, reading newspapers and smoking. It was bustling and bright, the opposite of the diner Edward Hopper painted, the postcard Vera kept in her macramé purse. Hopper painted with an "interior vastness," the postcard said, that made his diner the loneliest place on earth. His characters looked as if they had lost something but were too tired to go look for it. Vera believed they had stopped looking for intervention, divine or otherwise. What I thought about most, though, was what was beyond the frame: The characters stared past the borders of Hopper's brush to vistas only they could see. He created them but they had needs he could not fill. Vera said the genius of Hopper was making you wonder about what wasn't shown. I knew what she meant. It was better not to know everything, to keep a space the imagination could fill in, like the slivers of white on the page between letters and words.

Krispy Kreme evoked no such allusion. It was pale green, white, and dazzling. Its red letters stood in the sun like calligraphy copied from a book written by a monk.

Kurt came out with a dozen donuts, a cup of coffee, and an orange juice. He set the box on my lap, opened it, and lifted a chocolate-covered donut sprinkled with coconut. I chose a glazed. It was warm and sticky and light as spun cotton, and melted on my tongue quicker than communion. Kurt ate two more, one covered in crushed peanuts, the other a custard that drooled down his chin and onto his shirt. He laughed at the mess. He gunned the Impala and we screeched out of the parking lot with Krispy Kreme napkins whirling out of the backseat as if we were in a parade or had just won the World Series. The ocean was dead ahead. The waves lunged white and heavy on the shore and the spray kicked up rainbows in the sun. Kurt parked and sat on top of his seat and looked over the windshield to the water.

"The great beyond. Ships I've painted are out there making port-o-calls and emptying their bilge. My work sails around the world. I like knowing that. And after years they come back to be scraped of their barnacles and painted again. It's amazing, Jim, what the sea can do to something as hard and heavy as a ship."

Kurt opened his door. He took off his shoes and his custard-stained shirt, jogged across the blacktop, over the boardwalk, and across the sand, into the waves. I ate another donut and sat on the top of my seat, watching him. I felt like a king or a prince, lording over the world in a convertible, looking out at people on their blankets, all those lives and stories, the sounds of living tangled in the wind and blowing away like a ball of sound too knotted and intricate to decipher. I left Kurt to his waves and went up to Room 503. The bed was made, the Almond Joy wrapper and the roach of a joint were gone; the scents of the night before, gone; the carpet vacuumed, two white towels folded on the bathroom rack near a basket of soap, shampoo, and a rolled-up washcloth made to look like a bird. It was my room, but it was a new room, and tomorrow when I was gone, if we were still leaving tomorrow, the room would look the same for a new guest who wouldn't know that a boy from Philly touched for the first time a girl's breasts in this very place.

I went to 501 and knocked. Vera opened the door and pointed to a lipstick map on the mirror. The gun was on the bed, her purse was in shambles, and Vera was wrapped in a towel and wet from the shower, mascara dripping around her eyes like Alice Cooper.

"How was tennis, Jim? Did you beat that old man of yours? Where is he now? In the ocean I bet, washing off his sin. It's Sunday. A day for baptism. I got his note. I didn't worry, but I had to stay in the room. I sense the man is in this hotel or very close. I thought we were out of danger, but as I told you . . ."

She pointed to the lipstick map.

"It's pretty, don't you think? Quite specific, too. Streets in tangerine, escape routes in red. You, me, and Kurt will go over it later. We need to coordinate."

She sat on the bed so much smaller than when she'd told the tales of her past. Her shoulders were beaded with water, her hair flat and damp, lusterless. I thought of when we met in the diner, when

Vera spun into Philly drinking frozen lemonade vodkas and playing tennis with Kurt in the alley. I wished I could have kept that image of her, the way one cuts a picture to fit into a locket. But people won't let you do that to them.

Late the night before we left Philly, I came down to the kitchen and saw through the back door Vera sitting on Kurt's stoop. Her legs were pretzel-folded, her back straight; a candle shone before her in a glass beside two sticks of incense. She hummed, gathering light and smoke with her palms and washing them over her face. I wondered then what our neighbors would have thought looking out of their row-house windows and seeing Vera chanting and collecting candlelight as the *Inquirer*'s delivery trucks thunked bundles of papers on sidewalks and paperboys walked into the dawn with the world's news.

"Tell me a story, Vera. Something from far away."

"So many. Where to begin? I am a vagabond, Jim. I should have put all my experiences into songs and hymns. That's the best way to tell them. I'll think of a good story for later. Right now I've got to get out of this room."

She went into the bathroom and through the crack in the door I saw her towel drop on the floor and in the mirror I saw Vera's bare back. I turned away and sat on the bed by the gun. She came out of the bathroom wearing a long, gauzy white shirt over her black bikini, those big black sunglasses and that straw hat, looking like a movie star in hiding, an alabaster girl summoning courage to face the sun. I followed her into the elevator.

"Why is that radio downstairs always playing the Beach Boys? Jesus. They gotta change stations."

"Yup."

"Something classical, maybe."

The doors opened and we walked across the lobby — I didn't see Alice or Slim at the front desk — and out the door to the boardwalk. It was starting to feel like home. Vera scanned the beach and spotted

Kurt, tumbling through a wave, then rising and bending to catch his breath. Vera looked up and down the boardwalk, then behind her. She switched shoulders with her macramé purse and descended the stairs to the sand, hurrying toward Kurt, her straw hat blowing off, which I caught, and her white shirt tugged by the wind. She got to Kurt and hugged him, held on to him until he lifted her and spun her above the surf and she started laughing and crying and she whispered things into his ear and slid down his wet body so she could stand. She threw me her shirt and purse, but kept her sunglasses on as she and Kurt swam out over the surf to flat water. Kurt waved to me from out there, and I pretended it was a call for help, a plea from a distressed sailor who had tumbled off his ship. Vera looked like a bug in those big black glasses, chin skimming the water and her hair falling in straggles into the sea. I sat on the beach like a dog waiting to be walked. The sun was not too hot and every now and then a chalky cloud, tall and fat as a building, lumbered across the sky, throwing a shadow over the beach and chilling the air. I closed my eyes and listened, and I guess I must have fallen asleep; the next thing I saw was Kurt standing over me, dripping water on my face.

"Get up, boy," he said, laughing. "You think this is a vacation or something?"

Vera was still out beyond the waves. Kurt plunked in the sand.

"She okay?"

"Right now, yeah."

"She drew an escape map on the mirror. In lipstick."

Kurt half smiled. He sat like a breathing statue.

"There used to be slave ships out there, Jim. Not that long ago, either, in historical terms anyway. Could you imagine being a boy or a man chained for weeks, maybe months, in the bottom of a wooden ship? Chained to hundreds of others. What did they think at night, listening to the creaking of that big boat, wondering where in the hell they were going? Death and stink all around them."

Kurt let it stop there. He stared at the horizon. I imagined sea and shoal and forest and mountain rising in the blue-green of the New World. Not for those on the boat; theirs was a land of whips and ropes looped over trees, fields of cotton and tobacco and big pillared houses. It was hard for a white person to feel close to a black one. Even the black families on this beach, scattered dark splotches in the sand drinking out of coolers and building castles just like the white families next to them, seemed exotic, living in my world, but not exactly in it, as if there was another dimension, existing alongside mine but separated by a sheet of glass as clear and as impenetrable as a Krispy Kreme window. Everyone pretended, but sometimes make-believe was not enough, and that's when you felt bad about your white skin, how much it gave you, how much it took from others.

I had a black friend in Philly named Arenthal. He had a plug-in amplifier and Fender guitar and he wanted to be Jimi Hendrix; he wove leather headbands through his high-rise Afro and loved to show off a molar he chipped once while playing "The Star Spangled Banner" with his teeth. I met him one day after seeing him through Nut Johnson's telescope running at the school track. He was spindly, but fast. Nut and I went over and watched him, clicking and scrunching through the cinder in his spiked shoes that when he hit twenty yards turned to blur. I couldn't run that fast with three legs and a set of wheels. Nut's mother called him home for dinner, but I stayed, and Arenthal and I went for cherry sodas at a store between the white edges and black edges of North Philly. The *Inquirer* called such places "racial buffer zones" that kept the city from exploding. It was the make-believe world.

One night, I invited Arenthal to Nut's rooftop. He peered into the telescope, looked at me, amazed, and looked back. He aimed it as the stars and was so thrilled that he didn't step away at the crucial time — those heavenly minutes — when Nut wanted a glimpse at

Mrs. Romano. I knew what Arenthal felt, the first time you saw a star up close. He panned across black, sparkly space, pushing Nut, who was losing his patience, back and naming every star he saw. Funk. Otis. Martin. Malcolm. Shaft. Hendrix. Africa. He claimed them all. Nut said most stars already had names and were plotted with numbers and degrees, but Arenthal said he didn't care; he said everyone was entitled to as many stars as they wanted; no one could get to a star anyway, and no one person could own a million of them.

Sitting on a rooftop in the night with a black kid wasn't done often in my neighborhood and Nut and I, wanting to avoid questions and trouble and worse, never mentioned it. We snuck Arenthal down through Nut's narrow box of a house, past his sleeping parents, stepping over Wowser, the clawless ginger-colored cat, through the kitchen, and out the back door into the quiet alley, where Arenthal winked and sprinted home through the darkness.

"Goofy kid," said Nut.

"What do you mean?"

"Rather look at stars than tits."

Arenthal wasn't at the track the next day, or the one after that. Nut and I spotted him a few days later in the buffer zone with a cast on his right arm. Some guys in my neighborhood caught him and beat him the night he ran home from Nut's house. They held a knife to him and told him if he came back they'd cut him deep. They set his track shoes on fire. I went home and told Kurt (Dad) and he got upset and cursed. He gulped a beer on the stoop, talking to Mom, who sat below him, calming him, her head leaning against his leg. I listened through the curtain. I couldn't make out all the words, but later Kurt came into the kitchen and handed me thirty dollars and told me to give it to Arenthal for a new pair of track spikes. I had never seen that much money come out of Kurt's pocket at one time; even our special dinners at Howard Johnson's in New Jersey cost only fifteen dollars, which to Kurt was exorbitant, just like the electric and gas bills and the garbage collection fees that once a month gave him headaches and sent his checkbook flying off the table to the tune of words so foul that Mom told him he was mouthing the devil's aria.

What happened to Arenthal bothered Kurt for a long time and he kept asking me about him. I told him Arenthal bought new shoes and was running again at the track. He decided not to come over and look through Nut's telescope anymore, but we could say hi to each other and talk every now and then in the buffer zone. I saw him a few times, but then he vanished. One night, while I was sleeping, Kurt came into my room with a cassette player. He sat on the bed and pushed the button, and it was a voice I had heard snippets of in school over the years. I sat up and Kurt and I listened to Martin Luther King Jr.'s 1963 speech at the Lincoln Memorial; we just sat there, Kurt holding the tape player, listening as moonlight came through the window and the noises of the city fell distant and hushed. Kurt never mentioned that night or Arenthal again. He had a way of doing that, of getting so intense, so quietly feverish about something, that it burned a mark in you and you kept it as your own private thing. I asked Mom about it once and she said it often appeared that Kurt wasn't paying attention to things, that he'd drift away on the stoop or the couch with a whole other world going on in his mind, but that really Kurt paid attention to everything, and it was when you weren't paying attention that he'd surprise you with a new dress or a tape of Martin Luther King Jr. That's what had excited Mom most in life, wondering and waiting for Kurt's next revelation.

Vera returned from the sea. She sat next to Kurt and me on the sand, and if you were looking at us through Nut Johnson's telescope, you'd have thought we were a happy family. You would have given us a story: Ahhh isn't that nice, look how close they are, sitting on the beach wet and without towels enjoying the freedom of the day and the company of one another. Yes, you would have thought, the father must be a workingman; you can tell by the arc of his back and his taut, long muscles, and the boy is still growing, a budding astronomer or some other academic or bookwormish thing, and the mother, pale as winter sky in her black bikini, is protecting her pretty (they must be pretty) eyes behind dark pools of sunglasses. What's in her eyes, you would think. What does she see when she tousles her boy's hair and leans into her man, kissing and laughing with him in the sand and running down the beach, twirling in a gauzy white shirt, so gauzy as to be insubstantial, gauzy as smoke pulled apart by wind or by biplanes humming above the shore? You would have thought vacations never last long enough, and that in a better world they would never end; they would just go on and on like starlight and infinity, families at the beach, playing, swimming, and tanning in a buffer zone between birth and death. Then you'd pan the telescope to somebody else, make up another story, like counting cars on the highway or collecting postcards; it's all pretend dreams and mind games that get put away at the end of the week when the hotel bill is paid and the car is packed and the final glance is given to the rolling sea.

The maid fixed the bed and left new towels, but she did not touch the mirror in Room 501. Kurt studied Vera's lipstick escape map and told her we would follow the tangerine side street next to the hotel to the larger red road that led to the interstate. Vera stood beside him, biting her lower lip, her hair still dripping, and agreed, but not before laying out another route, which Kurt said was fine, but it would mean an extra two turns to the interstate. Too many wasted seconds; too much time for closing gaps. Vera shook her head. Kurt was appeasing the way a parent tricks a child into believing that the pillows and sheets on the floor are a magic castle of dungeons and spires and princesses. Vera went into the bathroom, turned on the shower, and started singing, not a particular song, just strands of chirpy notes and whistles. Kurt looked at me and laid out his own plan.

"When we were out swimming Vera thought the man from Marrakesh was below us in the depths. She clung to me, scared that she'd be snatched and pulled under. Then she calmed down as if a shark had drifted away. Even wanted to swim by herself. But these episodes are coming closer together. She needs help. I don't want to leave her alone. Dropping her off in a hospital and driving away wouldn't be right. I think we should play along awhile longer, pretend we're still on an adventure hiding from a bad man. We'll drive back to Philly and I'll try to get hold of her family. She said she was from Cleveland, remember? If we can't get them right away we'll call doctors and see what we should do. At least in Philly, if she's committed to an institution we can visit her. I want to believe her, but I can't anymore. Did you see her tracing the lipstick map, standing there, peering right through it, like a kid playing imaginary war in the alleys but thinking it was real."

"Did you see the pill bottles in her purse?"

"Yeah. They're empty. She was taking something, but the prescription was faded and I couldn't make out what it was."

"What if there really is a man? He's out there like she says, and that's what's driving her crazy, and every time she tries to convince someone, he's gone."

"I don't think so, Jim. That would be terrible if it were true."

"We don't know for certain, do we?"

"No, we don't. You want to believe it, don't you?"

"I'd rather believe that than the other. It's like when Mom died. I knew it. We went to the funeral home and I saw her next to the lilies, but I kept waiting for someone to come and tell me different.

"When do we leave?"

"Check out early tomorrow morning. We'll drive it in one day."

"What about the gun?"

"There are no bullets. We'll let her keep it."

Bad men. I've seen them on the news with numbers below their chins and eyes caught unaware. They appear right after dinner, hovering on the screen between six and six thirty, their lives and crimes compressed into a few lines, unless they did something spectacular, like killing housewives in bathrobes, boiling puppies, or robbing banks with toy guns. Kurt had known a few of them, union guys with drug habits and strange ideas about raising cash, like Leonard Lupo, who stormed a Moose Club with a bowie knife and a World War II grenade that blew up in his hand as he ran out the door, scattering money and blood into the air before bartender Mike Iaonne tied a rag around Leonard 's wrist, which looked like an orange that had been put through the squeezer, except that it was red, and carried him to the hospital on the corner, picking up bits of Leonard's blown-off hand on the way and calling the failed bandit a "dumbass and a fool beyond comprehension." I wondered if Kurt and I would be on the news; two guys in an Impala with a woman who disappeared, leaving only a scarf and a map on the backseat. The camera would pan and the scarf would lift in the breeze as two cops studied the map and Kurt and I stood near the hood of the Impala trying to explain that it began in the winter when a wife and a mother died in the Philly snow.

"A man from Marrakesh?" a cop would say. "What man from Marrakesh?"

Vera came out of the bathroom and she and Kurt went out. I studied Vera's lipstick lines on the mirror. We were there, invisible, wandering over clear glass. I traced. But where to go after the last red line opened up to the interstate? I-64. Streaking east and west, but beyond that, nothing but my reflection. I left 501. A whoosh of balcony air slammed the door behind me. A man pushing a stroller with a sleeping toddler smiled and went to the elevator and down to the beach. I stood in the hall, watching elevator numbers descend and rise, thinking about nothing and having no thought to move me, when the elevator opened and Alice stepped out with a box of soap and a tray of cut flowers.

"Ain't they pretty? Daddy found them at the Farm Fresh and wanted me to sprinkle a few in each room. Smell."

She lifted carnations, daisies, and a few she called irises.

"I'm going to put this one in your room. The petals are still perfect."

She kissed me on the cheek. She opened 503 and pulled me in, dropping flowers on the bed, holding me in daylight, showing me the pollen on her fingers, and saying that she couldn't stay but that she would be back. She handed me an iris and headed to the door, balancing her box of soap and flowers and singing "A Whiter Shade of Pale."

"Let's do something."

"I gotta put these flowers out. Daddy said to."

"I'll help."

"No."

"Let's go swimming."

"Boy, I gotta work. You go swimming. I'll see you later."

She walked away in her cutoffs and purple halter. How many colors did she have? I didn't want to swim. I took the elevator down. Slim was playing solitaire in the lobby, muttering to himself. A guy with white shorts and matching knee socks was reading the brochure about Indians, telling his wife, "Here's an interesting fact . . ." Kurt and Vera were talking to a man on the boardwalk. I went out the door toward them and saw the man had a Bible open on the railing and Kurt looked at me, saying in his eyes, *Jim, if you've got any sense, you'll keep on strolling.* I didn't. Bible pages lifted and riffled like white wings in the breeze. The young man was intense.

"The Lord saves," he said.

"Not everyone," said Vera.

"There are those who choose not to be delivered."

"I'm a Catholic," said Kurt.

"No harm. Catholics can be saved."

Kurt shisssed like he did whenever he missed an easy forehand.

"What about Hindus, Muslims, Buddhists? What about half the planet?" said Vera.

"Doomed."

"Doomed?"

"Only those who accept Christ . . ."

"You can't save me. Christ can't save me. You can't save anyone on this beach. You're a boy with a book of fables."

The guy's jaw tightened. Kurt looked to the sea. Vera stared at the guy, not angry, not dismissive, but with an open face: her soul challenging his. The man picked up the Bible, ran his fingers over its emblazoned gold cross. He didn't want to leave; he wanted a way in, but he had nothing. Jesus would have waited Vera out. He would have bent down, plucked something from the boardwalk, and spun a parable out of a sliver of wood.

The guy dipped his head and turned away, his back straightening as he walked toward another couple, his hair not even mussed by the breeze.

"Let's eat," said Vera.

"HoJo's?"

Vera laughed and kissed Kurt on the cheek.

"Where else, Kurt? Where else on this beautiful evening?"

Vera reached for my hand. The three of us walked down the boardwalk in the dusk, the first blossoms of neon sputtering and humming at the Fun Park, a child's voice wailing through the drop of a wooden roller coaster that dipped and clattered alongside us and shot back toward the sky. It was like it had been. Vera's worry had left her; the man from Marrakesh, there, but faint, at the edges. It was good to see her like that again. I studied her as we walked, her hand holding mine tight; her hair full around her, her face finally tan, as if in the course of the day she had slipped from one part of herself to another, like Superman, darting into a phone booth and coming out somebody else, but still with the hint, the discernible features of Clark Kent. You can't explain it; it's just that the better part returns and you wonder why it doesn't stay, it seems so perfect. Vera had that more than anybody, and I understood why Kurt wanted to be around her: not for love, he'd love only Mom, but for that moment of resurrection.

"Go win me a stuffed animal, Kurt. A small one."

He slapped a dollar down and hurled softballs at milk bottles. He slapped another down for me. We threw, balls exploding into cans, and the ones that missed, thunking against the tent. No animal. Two more dollars went down and Vera stood behind us licking cotton candy from her fingers. Kurt's first ball went high, knocking off only the top bottle, but mine was a direct strike at the middle, bottles flew and scattered in joyous ruckus. Vera threw down her cotton candy and clapped and the counter man handed me a kangaroo wearing boxing gloves, small just like Vera wanted, and she took it and kissed its face and I stood there feeling as if I had handed her the Holy Grail.

Kurt laughed and punched me in the arm and Vera said it was magnificent the way those bottles went flying. She put her arm around me and kissed me on the forehead. I was her hero; that's what she said. She held the kangaroo up and named him Sir Jim of the Strong Right Arm. We left the Fun Park for Howard Johnson's and Kurt, whom Vera had dubbed Kurt of the Wild Pitch, ordered his clams, Vera a Jell-O fruit salad with a tea, and a double cheeseburger and large Coke for me. Vera looked out the window once; her face tightened a bit, but only for a moment. Kurt paid the bill; we sat amid the change, dirty plates, and glasses watching the busboy, with his paper hat and hairnet, work his way toward us.

"I wonder what that young man is thinking," said Vera.

"He's daydreaming."

"How do you know?"

"By his face. Look at him. The only thing alive, barely alive, are his eyes, moving from dish to dish to fork. The rest of him is someplace else, someplace far away."

"Well, you're pretty smart, Mr. Wild Pitch."

"I do the same thing. It's how we stay sane."

"Who?"

"Workingmen."

"So all workingmen are out there daydreaming."

"That's right. Some are throwing pitches in the World Series. Some are rock stars. Some are on a date with a girl they'll never have. Some are designing spaceships, or waterbeds; some are praying and some are picking lottery numbers and imagining how they're going to spend it when it comes pouring in. It makes the hours go faster."

"What's your daydream, Kurt?" I said.

Kurt dipped his head and gave one of his sly smiles.

"The final game in the final set at Wimbledon. I'm up by a break. The grass is worn. The sky is clouding and everyone is worried about rain. The air cools. I'm out there with Jimmy Connors. Been on the court three hours and forty-five minutes. My hands are blistered. They sting. My knees ache; my toes are cramped. I'm serving. Jimmy's squatting in that fidgety nervous dance he does, left to right, left to right. I step to the baseline. Bounce the ball. A little chalk dust rises. I toss and spring from my coil, arcing, I feel the sweet spot. The ball goes off the racquet fast; it's going to curve and kick out, but Jimmy reads me and he's all over it. He returns at a sharp angle, but I get to it. The volley's on. The ball shooting back and forth. The crowd rises. They don't want it to end, and from my place on the grass I can feel thousands of eyes holding me.

"I hit a slice backhand to slow the pace. It kicks up funny on the grass. Jimmy mis-hits. The ball comes to me soft and high. I step in and drill it down the alley. Jimmy races to it but barely gets his racquet on it. I hear him grunt. The ball floats toward me high and at the net. I step in, not a thought in my brain, and put it away and see Jimmy racing for it, but it's beyond him and out of sight and Jimmy looks at me from across the net and then he drops his head and walks toward me. The crowd is going crazy, but Jimmy and I lean in and touch foreheads and find a piece of silence.

"When the prince or earl or whoever hands me the trophy cup, I'm struck by how light it is. It seemed so heavy when I had watched on TV as other champions lifted it. I take a shower. The blisters are raw and pink, the muscles are balled and tight, and the soreness settles in. But I stand there with the water rushing over me, feeling, I think, how God must want each of us to feel at least once on this earth."

A plate clattered at another table.

"I can see you running toward the ball, Kurt, your racquet back and waiting," said Vera.

Kurt lifted his soda.

"That daydream will get me through three or four cans of gray."

Vera leaned forward.

"You know what my daydream is, boys? To sleep one solid night without worrying that the man is getting closer. Just to breathe calmly and sleep, cool air running over my shoulders, like when I was a kid with the winter blanket falling away and me reaching for it, but still asleep, not waking."

"What's your daydream, Jim?"

I sat back.

Mine was of Mom, and lately, of Alice, but I didn't tell them. I must have blushed, though; Kurt and Vera pointed and laughed and I felt heat bleed across my face. I wanted Mom back. I wanted her to be waiting in our house after this adventure, but I knew she wouldn't be there and all the rooms would be empty. In my daydream

I whispered dictionary words to her, odd antecedents and unusual origins. She laughed at their sounds and meanings and said I was a smart boy of syllables and mischief; she told me this at the kitchen table when the late-afternoon autumn light was beyond the sink, retreating, leaving the kitchen dark, the white light of the rising moon far away down the street, when the neighborhood lingered in that in-between silence of dinners cooking and afternoon movies and men coming home and steam clinging to windows.

I looked at the busboy. He was a table away; dirty plates slipped through his hands like playing cards. He sweated through his hairnet and kept his head down; the world could have crumpled around him and he wouldn't have known. He had a faint mustache and sparse, coiled whiskers on his chin and jawline. His white busboy's shirt was stained with condiments and grease, the sleeves too long for his arms; his pants were black, his face pale. He seemed like candle wax come to life. A girl, a young woman actually, wearing cutoffs, a tank top, and flip-flops and carrying a baby on her hip walked in and kissed him on the cheek and stood in front of him. He didn't look at her for long. He reached into his pocket and handed her a few bills and she left, the baby waving its tiny, fleshy fingers at him. Kurt dropped a few extra quarters on the table and we slid out of our booth and back onto the boardwalk. We walked for an hour, not saying much, strolling to where the boardwalk ended at the dunes and the only lights were from ships in the black, black distance. Vera caught a chill and she walked back to the hotel between Kurt and me, each of us with an arm around her to warm her.

Room 503, my room, was full of flowers. I saw them when I creaked the door as Kurt and Vera passed to 501. I pushed the door open and light from the hall spilled into a room covered in daisies, roses, carnations, black-eyed Suzies, long-stemmed irises, and others I couldn't name in splashes of purples, reds, and yellows. They were thrown about as if tossed by wind and their scents held back the salt air of the beach. I stepped in, closed the door, and breathed them in. I turned on the TV and the flowers turned to silhouettes in the blue glow. I sat and smiled and watched the weatherman move the sun up the coast; farther north, Nova Scotia was lost in rain and fog and the weatherman noted that the Atlantic cold-water cod were running; it all tied in with Arctic air masses and deep, frigid currents. A guy with a lunatic's face and a cowboy hat popped up selling used cars and I turned the channel and saw a note on the mirror.

"Daddy ordered waaaaaay to many flowers from the Farm Fresh. Aren't they pretty?"

A girl's penmanship was a loopy thing of wonder. I read the note, put it back on the mirror, took it down and read it again, searching between words and letters for things not spelled out. I cried. I don't know why. It just came. Not long and sloppy, just real quiet; I held it deep in me and let it out a little bit at a time, the way you let the pressure hiss from a radiator.

I Dream of Jeannie came on. I propped a pillow and leaned back, covering myself in flowers. In the silences between the dialogue of Jeannie and Master, I heard the ocean. Jeannie crossed her arms and boinked — the sound like springs — and disappeared in a curl of smoke into her bottle. My face was tight from dried tears. I sat up and flowers fell and I went to the bathroom and put my face in a sink full of water. I dried and waited for Alice, peeking my head out the door every now and then to see if the elevator numbers were moving. I put my ear to the wall with 501, but I heard nothing, maybe a rustle, but their room was still.

I opened my dictionary, closed it. I went to the balcony and crossed the border from pollen to sea, the change dramatic; the flowers in the room turned to scentless beauty, as if under glass in a museum. I stepped back into the room and the flowers' scents filled me again, and the sea fell away as if it were not there. A knock. The slender rap of a girl's knuckles. I opened the door.

"You get my flowers?"

I laughed quietly and Alice stepped in. I closed the door. Alice knelt on the bed, flowers in her hair, counting petals in the dark. They floated like pieces of night.

"You're leaving tomorrow."

"Early."

"All the nice boys leave."

"How many?"

"A few, but no one got flowers. Only you. Kiss me once and lie down and let me sleep on your chest. We can't do more. If you were staying, maybe. I can't give my whole self to a boy who will be gone. But we can wake in the morning with a room full of flowers, and that'll be something you'll never forget."

We kissed. We kissed twice, even though she said only once. She gathered alongside me, her head was light. She traced my face with a finger.

"I'll draw you on paper later."

I closed my eyes. Lying there with Alice was good enough; I was curious about those places I had never been, but mostly I was happy just to feel her breathing in my arms on our private sea of flowers. She felt like a part of me, her skin mine, and I held her tight, not too tight to wake her but tight enough to claim her for the hours we had left. I played songs in my head and wondered about God looking down into all the rooms on earth, and what it'd be like when I was older lying in a different room with another girl, remembering Alice in the darkness of a new place. I watched the blowing curtain. The curtain in my room back in Philly rarely felt the breeze, the streets and alleys were so tight and narrow that the wind couldn't find our house; it blew past us to wider spaces beyond. The sounds, Alice's breathing, the waves, all went quiet, as if they were moving away from me and into the distance. I slept.

I don't know if I dreamed. I woke and Alice was still there on my chest; the dawn hadn't come, but the night was turning to gray dust and I could see blues, whites, yellows, and pinks flaming around me. I shut my eyes. A door in the hall slammed and the wall with 501 shook. I heard Vera, it seemed to be Vera, screaming not words but tangled indecipherable gasps. I jumped up from Alice and ran into the hall and saw Kurt standing at the door of 501 with a bucket of ice; cubes speckled the hallway as if he had run from the vending machines back to the room. He must have heard her scream, too. He saw me and rolled his eyes. Vera's screeches came through the door. Kurt reached for the knob and slowly opened 501. I heard a pop and saw Kurt's ice skip out of the bucket and fly around him like tiny, clear planets. Kurt's body jolted back and he looked down and dropped the bucket and then stepped wobbly across the threshold. I heard another pop and glass break. I ran and saw Kurt lying on the carpet, two paintbrush strokes of blood widening from him, one near his chest and the other at his thigh.

Vera was standing on the bed in underpants and no shirt, the silver gun heavy and smoking near her breasts. She was crying and shaking and screaming, "The man! The man!" The room smelled like the scene of a toy cap-gun fight; the scent of gunpowder, but deep in it a musky, sweet tang. Vera's lipstick mirror map was shattered and the TV screen was static with the color of salt and pepper. I got down next to Kurt. His blood warmed my knees. All his muscles were still. His eyes were open as if examining the fallen galaxy of ice around him. I lay beside him and held him and asked him not to go.

"Kurt, please stay." I kept saying please like I did when I was a child trying to get something from him he didn't want to give. I gripped his hand and looked into his face, sideways and scrunched on the carpet. He squeezed my hand and tried to say something, but the word stopped, half formed in his mouth. His eyes closed like they did when he'd stand on our stoop after work and drink his beer before dinner. I didn't want to take my face off the carpet.

I wanted to stay staring at him, holding him; I wanted to go where he was going and to wait for that frozen word to be released from his mouth. He was about to tell me something, something I needed to know.

Alice and Slim stood in the doorway. Vera stayed on the bed and dropped the gun to her side, her head tilted down, eyes looking through ragged hair, her body trembling.

"He was here. He was here. When Kurt went to get ice he snuck in and slammed the door and when Kurt came back he disappeared out the door just as I fired. I wanted to kill him. I wanted to end it. But, oh, Jim, I shot Kurt. He got away, down the hall and across the beach. I'm sure. I told you he was here, so close, always so close. I wanted to kill him, but look what I've done, Jim. Look what he's made me do."

She stepped off the bed and fell to her knees and slid the gun toward the bathroom. She crawled to Kurt and me. She lay with us. She stroked Kurt's hair and whispered to him; whispering and whispering, filling Kurt's ear with words but no stories. Her sounds were brittle, breaking in the air around her. I wanted to push her away but I didn't want to let go of Kurt. She was no longer that girl we met in the Philly diner. Curled and half naked and streaked with Kurt's blood, Vera was a strange finger painting, a refugee from a faraway place. She stopped whispering. She sobbed in long silent shakes along Kurt's body. She kissed his forehead. I couldn't look at her. I closed my eyes. I kept my hand in Kurt's and felt his calluses and saw him playing tennis, not with Jimmy Connors but with me, the two of us hitting in one of those rich suburbs outside Philly. I pressed closer to him, my nose touching his nose like I did when I was little and snuck into his and Mom's room and lay between them and listened to their breathing.

I waited to feel his breath, but nothing came, and from far off I heard squawking radios and men talking. They moved closer and I opened my eyes and saw shoes appearing around me, black shoes so shiny I could see my reflection next to Kurt. I closed my eyes again and held Kurt, trying to get us back to that tennis court, where I chased one of his down-the-line shots, lunging for it and finding the racquet's sweet spot, my return flying back at such an angle that all Kurt could do was watch the ball speed past him, and then look across the net to me as if I had done something miraculous.

The black shoes closed in and I felt hands pull me away from Kurt. I didn't let go but one of the men pried my fingers from Kurt's, and the men lifted me and it seemed I was floating. When they put me on the ground, I dove back and held Kurt again. Tighter. The men peeled me away and I cursed them. They sat Vera in a chair and draped her in a blanket, and she almost disappeared; a cop drew chalk marks on the carpet and another one slid the gun into a plastic bag the way I had seen them do in the movies. It all moved slowly as if everything was beating with half a heart, and scrapes and clicks and noises warbled in my ears like trapped birds. Alice hugged me and stepped away. The men held my arms and led me down the hallway. I squirmed to get back to Kurt but they were too strong. I heard the elevator ping and felt melting ice beneath my feet as I turned into Room 503. It was full of morning light and flowers left too long without water.

seventeen

"That's where it ends, James. You in that room full of flowers."

"Do you know what happened next?"

"Yes. Your life happened, James. From that day till now. Thirty-nine years of life."

"Kurt died."

"Yes."

"Vera?"

"I don't want to speak of her."

"Where is Kurt buried?"

"You've been there. In Philly near your mother, not far from the shipyards."

"I loved him."

"Yes."

I am sitting in a chair looking out a window in a room that feels like a hotel. It's night. I see the white foam of a wave in the distance and a man's reflection in the window. His head moves when mine does; his hands, too. He is sitting next to another reflection. A lady with a slender neck peers through the window to the sea, a wineglass at her lips. It seems the two reflections are characters in a pantomime or movie, their lives playing in a window illuminated in the sand. The lady's hand moves. She puts the wineglass down, stands, takes a step, and sits on the man's lap, on my lap. The man in the window is gone, covered by the lady, like a blanket or a shawl.

"I'm thinking of taking a trip to Poland, James. To visit where I came from. See old faces."

She kisses me on the forehead. She is light, warm. Her hair smells of sea and herbs.

"Do you remember your first time at the National Museum in Warsaw, James?"

I don't remember anything.

"It was, maybe, 1990, sometime shortly after the Wall fell. We went to the ground-floor exhibit of Christian iconography. Remember? You were struck by the suffering. There were Christs in marble, carved in wood, painted; images of a twisted, agonized Savior through the centuries. Crowns of thorns and tears of blood collected by angels with goblets. It was, you said, like a still-life horror movie. Image after image, everywhere you turned. You didn't get it, though. I told you that nobody suffers for their faith like the Poles. The torment of that broken Christ is our national metaphor. We endured through history and then we took His suffering and made it ours. Our strength . . ."

The lady's words are soft in my ears. Her voice is cracked with a husk, like a radio voice. It is lulling. I feel the hairs on my arm rise as she whispers.

"We left the museum and went walking through downtown Warsaw. We came upon the granite soldiers, so big and blocky. They stood on the corner. Stone monsters, you said. But they were not. The memorial flame lit them in the night. And don't you remember the snow falling around us, and we kissed among the big stone men and their helmets and guns? You said right then that you loved me and we kissed and drank wine in a café until they kicked us out and we walked to our hotel through a deep snow."

The lady stands.

"You said you loved me, James. For the first time, in the snow all those years ago."

She pours wine. She sits in the empty chair; there are two reflections in the window. Snow is the last word I hear. The image she

174

gave me is gone. Starting at the center and crumbling toward the edges, like when Kurt and I watched *Bonanza* and the flame seared through the middle of the Cartwright map and raced to the corners, that's how my mind loses things — in burning, black, widening holes. I try to concentrate, but neither picture nor memory survives. Only Kurt and Vera. Who is this lady? Should I run into the night toward the curl of the wave? No, I will sit. It is pleasant. The chair is comfortable. The lady's voice is pretty; there's a movie in the window.

"How many stories have you written, James?"

She asked this before. I can't say for sure, but it seems so. I must be a writer.

"A journalist," she corrects.

She keeps talking. She is a tour guide. She knows stories from all over the world, and in each of them I have a place, I think, but I can't hold the stories for long, and I see in her face that she is trying to will something, to convince me into belief, and I'd like to help her, because she is nice and has a pretty voice, actually all of her is pretty, but I cannot, and I can see in her eyes that I am disappointing her, but her eyes are tender, so very blue and tender. She pours more wine.

"What kind of child would we have had, James? I often think of this. What would have happened that night under that bright moon in Tunisia if I hadn't bled in that taxi and lost it? I felt it leave me, James, like a spirit from a room. I wonder what he or she would have become, raised by two nomads like us."

The lady stops talking. It's quiet. I look in the window, but in the illumination there are no tears like the ones I see when I turn toward the lady. That's how movies are. Kurt said movies seemed like real life but were really only tricks of light. Wind rattles the window; the reflections shimmy like pictures on water.

The lady turns toward me. She holds my hand. She rubs it with both her hands, pressing my palms and sliding down my fingers.

She says I used to have carpal tunnel from typing so much and at the end of workdays we'd sit in our apartment in New York and look over the river and she'd massage my hands and wrists as we watched lights harden in the dusk. Then we'd go out for dinner. She says we ate mostly Chinese and Italian, but that our favorite place was an Ethiopian restaurant hidden on a cross street up by Columbia University. We went to jazz clubs and sometimes, with friends, out to Long Island in autumn to see the leaves change and houses reel in their awnings and board up their windows for winter. She said life was good. Clever conversations and faces around tables chattering about everything from Bratislava to Khartoum, and on Sunday afternoons a long walk along the river and holding hands watching a black-and-white movie in a small cinema, where the popcorn man ran the projector and scents of dampness and perfume lingered in thick red seats. Those cinemas were her favorite places in New York; the old world lived in them, stories and tales of great European directors composed in shades of gray, full of meaning, but disappearing like ash when we walked home in the afternoon drizzle. This life sounds good — the parts of it, anyway, that don't evaporate as soon as she recites them.

Once, she says, I was mugged late one Saturday night on my way back home with the Sunday paper, still warm with news, like bread from the oven. One man pulled a gun, another a knife. The man with the knife hit me and stabbed my shoulder, but my coat was thick and the knife only pricked a muscle. The one with the gun grabbed my wallet and they both ran, but the man with the gun was not paying attention and was hit by a taxi when he crossed the street. My wallet went flying out of his hand, business and credit cards fluttering in the night. The man was not dead. He rose from the pavement and limped away, his pants torn and bloody. The taxi driver checked his hood. I picked up my wallet and went home with the paper and the lady put alcohol on my cut. It stung and we made love because I was alive.

"After all the wars you'd covered, James, to die in a mugging would have been cruel."

She sips her wine.

"Actually, it would have been the kind of story you would've liked to have written."

She stands and walks to the bathroom. I hear water and the scrape of shower curtain rings. I stand and go to the window. I try to open it, but it is painted shut and I get my coat and hat and walk out of the room. I don't know where I'm going, but I want to be outside.

I follow the long corridor to the red EXIT sign and push open the door, go down a flight of outside stairs, and find myself on the boardwalk. There's nowhere really to go; it's black and lonely out here, but I don't mind. I walk and listen to the sea. The wind is strong. I gulp cold air and my eyes water and I feel happy, but I don't know why. I have no details out of which to make happiness. I have one stretch of memory, that's it, and although most of that stretch is good, the ending is not, but I'm on this boardwalk in the night feeling happy and not knowing why. Instinct. Maybe the body remembers things the mind forgets. I don't know. I just want to be joyous at this moment, careless as a blank and windblown page.

The boardwalk disappears and I am in the dunes, the sounds of tall grass and wind rattle and whistle in my ears. In the fleeting sense that I know myself, I feel like an explorer in uncharted country, eyes in the black looking at me from the sea, and from way down the beach, a pier lit to its bones by a moon as intricate as a face. I feel as if I'm in a soothing tumult, so much going on at the edges, but inside, a quiet, like a cave in a forest storm or after those stickball games with Kurt, when he and I sat on the stoop while the other boys walked home, a dispersing army of banter and jokes. I sit in the sand and look at the black sea and its thread-like curls of white. I feel tears on my face, loping down my cheeks and off my chin. Where they're coming from, I don't know. Memory has taken my stories; how can

I have tears? But they're there, sticky as salt air. I let them be. I sit, but I don't know for how long; waves are not good for keeping time, they all look the same, unless I am tricked and I'm only seeing one wave over and over again. A voice.

"James. James!"

I see nothing.

"James!"

It comes closer.

"James."

A lady in a white bathrobe carrying a blanket comes around a dune toward me. Her hair is aslant in the wind, but she walks steady in the sand. She seems to float. She drops on her knees before me, puts a hand to my cheek, and I think this has happened before but I can't be sure. Her hand is warm; her thumbs rim my eyes, and she is collecting my tears.

"James. I'm Eva. Where have you been? You left the room, James. You can't do that. You can't wander off. What if I couldn't find you? Don't do that again, please. I was sick. I thought you drowned. No more walking off. Promise."

I feel like a child.

"I went in the bathroom to take a shower. Just for a second. Were you scared? Did you feel alone?"

"No. I am watching waves."

She kneels behind me, wraps her arms around me, and puts her head on my shoulder.

"Don't wander again please, James."

The air is still.

"I've told you all our stories but one, James. Would you like to hear it here on the beach? It's cold, but I have this blanket and if we sit together, we'll be warm."

"Let's stay."

She whispers in my ear. It was in Egypt. I had come from covering the war in Iraq and we met in Cairo and flew to Luxor. We were to take a boat down the Nile, through the desert and the Delta, all the way to Alexandria where the river opened to the sea. It was her idea. In Poland, when she was a child, her favorite book was a book of maps, and her favorite map was of the great river running snake-like past pyramids and cities of the dead.

We boarded a thirty-foot wooden sailboat, an old, sturdy thing with bleached wood and sails that were once white but had turned to the color of dust. The captain wore a turban and tunic. He walked barefoot on the deck, his face dark and wrinkled but brightened by a spray of white stubble. His son was second mate, a chubby, round-faced boy with cut hands and rope burns on his wrists. He made tea on the stern and blew flies off sugar cubes.

We left, gliding north in October. The sails filled. The boat moved slowly and she and I sat on the deck in ball caps and sunglasses, legs stretched out reading books and watching farmers and women in colorful tunics balance stacked bread and jugs on their veiled heads on the shore. I told her about the war, but not much, just a few stories of firefights and the craters and bloodied markets left by suicide bombers, and the way, after one explosion, hundreds of watermelons burst open like a garden of wet, pink flowers in the sun.

She had flown over from our apartment in New York. The Nile trip was to be an adventure before I began another book. Apparently, I've written books. How can this be? No memory of all those words.

She says we'd lie on the deck and feel the sun, which was strong but not too hot, and listen to the boy's propane flame and to the captain string sails, and along the shore we'd hear the call to prayer from villages, and she'd close her eyes and pretend she was Cleopatra; that's how ancient it seemed with the wooden boat creaking through the slow current.

"Don't you remember that, James? That feeling. That sense of timelessness that we never felt in Europe."

At night we made love in our cabin, still, moving only when a breeze ruffled the sails. We were as quiet as spirits, holding each other and listening to the captain and his son on deck speaking their language beneath the stars. One of the best things about us was how we made love, and how, no matter where we were, we found a way.

The captain brought the boat to shore in the mornings, and we'd eat round bread and eggs and wander into villages. Children danced around us, women looked down, and men smiled on their way to the fields, staring at Eva's unveiled hair and the skin on her arms beneath her pushed-up sleeves. We sailed around the bend at Qena and past El Manshah and Asyut, where the Eastern Desert stretched toward the Sinai, and seashells millions of years old shone like curled pearls in the sand. One morning we walked through a canyon, dry, the colors of parchment and bone, and climbed a cliff to the rim of blue sky, where we sat and drank wine — a very bad Egyptian one — in the shade of a crevice as if we were hiding from the world. The wind through the crevice made the rocks speak, or so we imagined. We sat there for hours, kissing and talking, perhaps a little drunk, looking through the ragged gash of rock to the cloudless sky. We were tan and started to smell of the desert and the marshes, and for the first time in a long while we were free.

"Life quieted, James."

She read Rumi and other Sufi poets and she would quote verse in the dusk as we sailed north.

"I wish you could remember. How can you forget that buried desert room we wandered into painted with hieroglyphs and owls and scorpions? Walls of stories, James. You were amazed. You ran your fingers over all those tiny, etched pictures. You copied some in your notebook. We were explorers."

The lady whispers in my ear; I don't remember, but I listen. We stopped near Zawyet el Amway late one afternoon. The captain took on supplies and said we'd spend the night on shore. He gave us an old canvas tent and some food and pointed us down a dirt road that after about two miles stopped at an oasis. Nobody was there. The desert air was cooling so we collected wood and brush and made a fire. The wood burned hot but quickly, needing to be fed for an hour until a bed of embers glowed in the circled rocks. We put the tent up; there was no wind and when night came, the stars laid out white across the sky. We drank wine and ate chocolate and sat close against the chill.

She says the conversation went like this:

"Are you scared?"

"No."

"It's black and empty."

"We're Bedouins. We have a tent and a fire."

"It's all we need, isn't it?"

"And that extra bottle of wine."

"Kiss me."

"Let's never go back. Let's just live by this oasis."

"Could we do that?"

"I think we could."

"Can you farm?"

"I'm more of a shepherd."

The lady says we heard footsteps in the night; soft, sandals through sand. A man appeared at the edge of the fire. He wore a tunic with a thick-spun blue scarf around his neck and shoulders. He had a drawn, brown face and a gray-black beard that spilled over the scarf; his hair was cut short and he wore a white skullcap. He bent and dipped his hands in the water and washed his face. He slipped off his sandals and splashed his feet. He unspooled his scarf and dried himself. He laid the scarf in the sand and knelt prostrate. He prayed. It was soothing, like a strange, delicate insect singing. He finished and stood. He coiled the scarf around himself and walked closer to the fire and sat. An ember popped and sparks flew around him like fireflies and he seemed like a man who had wandered in from centuries ago.

"A good fire. You will be warm through the night."

"I hope so. It's too dark to find any more wood."

"Are you traveling?"

"I am on a pilgrimage."

"To Mecca?"

"A private pilgrimage. A quiet one."

"We're on something similar."

"To be alone in the world."

"Are you Egyptian?"

"I was born farther south near Sudan."

"Are you a cleric?"

"Just a man with his God. I am Mahmoud. May I rest by your fire?"

"Please."

The man closed his eyes and opened his palms to the embers, smiling as the heat went through him. He was from a tribal family, but he left when he was young, urged and financed by a rich cousin from Tunisia to study in religious schools in Cairo and Alexandria. He memorized the Bible and the Koran and traveled through Europe, hitchhiking and sleeping in mosques and basements of Arab booksellers in Geneva and Berlin. He wasn't on a spiritual journey, although he said he was moved by the German romantics and their philosophies on nature, so different from the teachings of Islam, which had turned to God because the desert gave little repose. He thought about that, how landscape, the earth, makes our God. His journey opened a door; he didn't call it a revelation, but he learned something about himself, the way a serial killer or a chess master realizes early on that the voice within is slightly askew.

He woke one day with a gift. He could see into people's lives, not just what had happened, but what was to come. Every person he met was a character with their story written on their skin and in their eyes, invisible to everyone but him. He knew when they were born, when and how they would die; he knew them like bugs suspended on pins, and he could see all this with only a glance. How they took, how they loved, and what things they kept hidden.

He felt like a voyeur or a mad scientist peeking into diaries, but he wasn't peeking, and sometimes he would turn away, but when he looked back, the scroll spun again and the hidden things, the things nobody should know about another, become known to him, as if angels and demons whispered in his ears from white and black books. We listened to the man, both of us thinking it was an intricate pitch to tell our fortunes for money.

"It was the perfect setting, James. We were two miles from the boat with our tent and fire in the desert. We even thought this man Mahmoud was a relative of the captain's and that's why the captain had sent us to the oasis, so we could be entranced in the night and pay — not much, it's never really too much — to have stories told beneath the stars. Oh, James, we thought, without saying a word to each other, what a great seduction it was. Even his voice, don't you remember that slow, ancient rasp?"

He did not like the comparison to a fortune-teller. He had seen, like he did with us, suspicion in the eyes of people he confided in, and he grew to accept this after thinking one day how odd his gift must sound to those without it. He stopped confiding. He stopped wanting to know people's stories; he sought quiet and blank pages. Secrets, he said, were a burden, a dreary weight. He returned to the desert and found peace amid the bone-rock and sand. He kept to himself; he used the analogy of John the Baptist wandering with grasshoppers and honey on the fringes among the stones. Those he did meet were villagers or Bedouins whose hidden things were little different from the things they openly carried. There were a few tourists who glowed with angst and hidden things, huddled in their encampments until daybreak when jeeps carried them to the next spot on the map.

"Imagine," said the man, "standing in line at Burger King and knowing what the man before you would order even before he knew. You'd be surprised at how many people, right to the moment they step to the silver counter, are wrestling between a single or double cheeseburger. The torment."

He laughed at this story.

"What intrigued me most," said Mahmoud, "was the Catholic act of confession. In that little wooden box is where hidden things are to be revealed and forgiven. But hidden things are only halfway told. Even there, with the priest behind his scrim, people can't utter who they are. They can't tell their wives, their husbands, their children. It made me sad. We do not know anybody. We are all icebergs. The gist of us buried."

"But knowing those stories, could you have helped?"

"I am not a healer. I am a cipher."

The lady and I played along with Mahmoud, indulging him around the fire.

"But a man who would commit suicide," said the lady. "A child running in front of a car. A boy going off to war to be killed. Did you even want to stop that? To intervene? To misplace a second or a minute in someone's life, diverting them in another direction, away from dangers or pain."

"That would make me God. I am not Him."

"But you have power to see."

"It is a burden, not a power."

"Is there goodness?"

"Yes. All that's hidden is not bad."

"Can you read your own story?"

"No. I find that funny. Very curious, actually. I know the lives and hidden things of all but my own. That is God's way, I suppose;

one gift denies another. I meditate. I pray before Him, hoping to gather myself and see my identity in His mystery. But it doesn't come. There is a wall. My life's work now is to break that wall."

"Do you see our stories across the fire."

"Yes."

"Are we happy?"

"You know you are."

Mahmoud curled by the fire that night and when we awoke, he was gone, and for a moment we thought he had been a dream, but he had left his blue scarf coiled by the circled rocks and ash. We didn't know what to think, she says. Was he a talisman, a trick of the desert? When we asked the boat captain later, he shrugged with the slice of a smile as if he knew but wouldn't say.

I started to forget things in the months after we left Egypt, little annoying things: keys, leaving hot water running, losing places in books, looking confused in the morning, walking away from a laptop in an airport lounge. We joked that I would forget my nose if it wasn't attached. It got worse. I'd wander off, and once I rode the subway all day and ended up in a Brooklyn church sitting in a confessional with no priest. The organist asked for my wallet and called the lady to bring me home. There were many stories like this and one day the lady gave me a bracelet engraved with our address and phone number. I misplaced it.

It is dark, but there is light far off. The lady in the bathrobe talks in my ear, her arms holding me from behind; we sit in the sand, watching the thread of waves. The air is unstirred, cold. Her words, her breath, warm my skin. It is a good place to be, sitting with this lady, whom I don't know, but who keeps talking as if we are one. She means no harm; her stories live inside me, briefly, then blow away. I know enough to know this. She tells me about a man, Mahmoud, and how the Nile begins in Rwanda and flows north, absorbing tributaries and canals, widening in the delta, turning the desert fertile before spilling into the sea. The lady rises and stands before me. She holds out her hands, so white in the night.

"C'mon, James. It will be dawn in a few hours. We need to sleep before I take you back."

I grab her hands and rise. We walk between two dunes and to the boardwalk. Her robe is bright against the darkness. We enter a hotel, a slight man in a green jacket with gold buttons tips his head and smiles. Down a hall, into a room. The bathroom light is on, but the rest of the room is dark. I stand at the bed looking out the window. I see a reflection. A lady's hands come and take off my jacket, my shirt, my pants, and the colors in the reflection fade to the pale of a naked man who seems to be looking in from the beach, but his hands move when mine do, and the lady takes off her robe and stands in front of me; her back reflected in the window. She holds me and we ease into the bed. The lady doesn't speak; she lies beside me, and I feel her finger move over my forehead, down my nose, across my lips, over my chin.

"I am tracing you, James."

I have been here before, but I can't say when. Her touch, this light between night and dawn, I know them, the picture of the schooner on the wall, the desk beneath the mirror. I know them, but from where and when? The lady traces and kisses me. I close my eyes. She breathes into my ear, kisses my neck; she moves on top of me and I feel how light she is. She reaches down. I am inside of her. Warm. Like home. But I have only one home, years and years behind; I suppose it exists no longer and I don't know where home is now, maybe this room; I don't know. The lady sits up; she is warm but like a statue, not moving; she pulls my hands to her breasts and then up to her face; her face is in my hands; she is not moving; she is a statue, but so warm, the lightness of her being centered on me. I feel her love, but I don't know her name. The lady. She is like a statue, yes, but like a bird, too, perched, waiting.

"James."

I am James.

"Come back."

The statue moves. The bird aflight. I watch her; a shadow, a moving shadow taking color, white, an amber white, gathering in the dying darkness. I can't make her out, her hair is swaying, blocking her face, then revealing it, then disguising it again; she is older than Alice, Alice with the flowers, a room full of flowers at the beach, but the lady is not Alice; she is older like me, but I see, I think I see, how she must have looked younger; I think I saw this lady years ago, somewhere in the snow, perhaps on a city street, maybe I passed her in a city a lifetime ago, but where? To what cities have I been? I know her. She is making love to me. One doesn't make love with strangers, but I don't know anymore, what is strange and what is not, I just lie here, watching her over me, as if she wants to capture me and bring me back to some place in the light, and the light is filling the room, and all the blurry things are taking shape, except for me and this lady; we are in the light, but she is unknown to me, although I hear her say:

"James. James."

Whispers in a cracked voice. A voice rich, resonant with tone, a smoker's voice.

"James."

"Yes."

"Are you back?"

"I don't think so."

"What's my name?"

"I don't know but I feel we have met."

"Where?"

"I don't know. There are no distinctions. Inside of me, nothing is distinct. Do you understand?"

"Sometimes when we make love you come all the way back."

"Tell me."

The lady slides alongside me, still. I hear her breathing and feel her tears, and between my neck and shoulder there is soothing warmth.

"It's funny in a way, James. I am Eva from Poland. That's what I keep telling you, and it makes me feel like years ago when I was a professor in Warsaw and the police suspected me of spying. They put me in a room. They kept asking me questions and I kept giving them answers, but they didn't believe me. They looked at me blank, like you."

"Were you a spy?"

"For a while, right before the world changed."

"Was I a spy?"

"No. But you lived like one."

"Do you love me?"

"Yes, James, very much."

The lady stands naked in the light. Her body has no scars; it is the color of pigment, white, pink, like the polished shells they sell at souvenir shops, and another color, a shade of something deeper.

"See, James, I am much older than when we first met. The lines don't hold so taut anymore, but I try. Can you look into me, look through me to the girl you met? Remember."

She reaches for my hand. I sit on the edge of the bed in front of her. I wrap my arms around her; my head balanced beneath her breasts. I hear her heart, and she strokes my hair, and I don't remember a thing, but I hold her not wanting to let go.

"We started every morning like this. I would get out of bed first. You were always groggy, and I'd come around and pull you up and you'd slump into me and hold me just like this, and then you'd gradually stir and we'd make love in the morning, before, as you said, the noises of the day found us."

"If that happened, I was lucky."

"You were."

She kisses me on the head and turns toward the bathroom; a fish escaping through a net. She half closes the door.

"Don't wander off again. I'll be right out."

I sit naked on the bed, listening to the shower, watching steam curl up the mirror. My arms are thin, shapeless; I think I was once stronger. I see raised veins and slackened skin where muscle must have been. I flex my bicep; a slab rises in a sad arc. I was a boxer once. No, Kurt was the boxer. He had the thick arms and biceps, dancing in our basement and slapping that bag, his sweat spraying onto the blackened beams that held up the house. I smile at the thwack, thwack, thwack of Kurt's gloved fist against the leather. I stand and shadowbox like Kurt taught me, exhaling and throwing fists, a naked man fighting the air. I laugh. The rings on the shower curtain scrape; the lady, wet like a sheen, an ice statue melting, wraps a towel around herself and walks to me.

"What are you doing?"

"Boxing."

She rolls her eyes.

"Your turn."

I am alone in the shower, the curtain, like the shade in a confessional, is pulled but I can see the lady, like I used to see Fr. Heaney. I peek out through a crack in the curtain. She is wiping steam off the mirror and putting on makeup. She looks as if she's crying, but that might be the steam and the water. I wash my face and step out and dry myself. She is dressing. I know I have watched this before; her back bent, I see the side of her breast, the bra rising over it, an arm through a strap and the breast hides, lost in black lace like a crescent moon slipping into clouds. Women do this, I think, when they dress. Mom did it. Vera, too. And this lady. They turn their backs like in paintings, images in profile with hair falling over their shoulders, their chins dipping, legs lifting into stockings, like dancers backstage, and breasts hidden the way Mrs. Romano's breasts were silhouette and mystery in Nut Johnson's telescope. Men don't dress pretty.

"Time to get you back, James."

"Where?"

"The place you live. Philly."

A man with a green hat and gold buttons waves good-bye. The car is cold. I watch the waves out the window. No one is on the beach; we turn and the ocean is gone, and we pass under a string of lights to the edge of town where a green sign points to the expressway and the lady shifts into fifth gear and we race up the ramp through a gray morning with a crack of sun in the distance.

"All the stories have been told, James. There are no more."

She reaches down and holds my hand; wind is whistling and it feels like we are flying. We cross the bridge into Philly. I know these streets, not by name anymore, but I know them.

"I feel lost, too, James. In the strangest way. Years spent translating for you. Changing words from one language into another. I was a magician. Your rhythms became mine. Your words became mine and the words I gave you back became yours. But now you are not here and all words mean nothing. You are not you and because of that I am not me."

We stop in front of a brick building with white pillars, ivy, and a small gabled roof over the entrance. The windows have shutters; a statue of the Madonna stands in a garden. There is rust at her feet. The lady shuts off the car but doesn't move. She stares through the windshield; she looks at me and back to the windshield. The car creaks, the sound of oil cooling against engine metal. Tick. Tick. Tick. The lady turns toward me, takes my face in her hands, and kisses me on the forehead. She runs two fingers through my hair. I feel special but I don't know why. The lady gets out and opens the trunk. I get out, too. She hands me a small zippered bag.

"I'm going to Poland for a while. Remember, I told you? Of course, you don't. You've stopped remembering, haven't you?"

"I remember Kurt and Vera."

"I know. They are your only story. A man who once wrote thousands of stories has one left. Why does it have to be that one?"

She is crying.

"I feel you love me, but I'm sorry I don't know why."

"What's my name? Say it, James. Please, just once."

I look down. She holds me near the side of the car; the morning is gray and the streets are slick, shiny almost, with autumn frost, and children, off-balance with book bags, run toward a school bus and a crossing guard holds up a stop sign and the world seems to stop as the children step onto the bus and the lady keeps holding me, pressing into me hard, and the bus doors close and the stop sign comes down and the crossing guard walks to the corner and lights a cigarette and I think I see snow in the distance, just a few flakes over a car, and then whirling toward me, but they disappear or maybe they weren't there at all. My eyes are blurry from the cold and the lady lets go of me and gets into the car and I am standing alone with a small zippered bag in my hands and the lady rolls down the window and I see tears on her face and I think she was pretty when she was young because she's so pretty now and it bothers me that I should know her name but I don't; the engine starts and the lady waves for me to come closer and she whispers to me. Her hands reach out the window. I bend down; her fingers run through my hair. She pulls me close. I feel her breath in my ear.

"I am Eva, James. I was with you when the world changed."

She releases me. She rolls the window up and drives away, down a street shiny with autumn frost.

A woman in a coat and white hat steps beside me.

eighteen

I am the woman in white. James stands on the curb with his overnight bag as if he's waiting at the wrong bus stop. It makes me sad. I take his arm. His eyes are fixed on Eva's red car; she turns and is gone, leaving only a wisp of tailpipe smoke at the corner by the market she often stops at to buy cigarettes on her way back to New York. Not today. She had called me earlier to say she was going away and wouldn't be seeing James for a while. That's not like Eva, but I understand, and maybe she'll be back or maybe it'll be just James and me from now on. She loves him, so I have hope, but sometimes hope is hard. I nudge James and smile at him. Vacant. It's cold and Christmas decorations will be up soon — tinsel strung, blown-up Santas, snowmen painted on windows. I'm a simple wreath girl; the world's full of too much sparkle as it is.

I have to shop for James, though. Last year I bought him one of those little iPod Shuffle things and had a friend's son download the *White Album* on it. James liked it. I think he did. I'd better get him inside. We walk up the stairs, take two lefts, and follow the long hallway to his room. I take off my coat so he can see my white uniform and he looks at me as if he thinks he has seen me before. He does this every day; white is soothing. The color of angels.

I will spend the weekend with James. It's all planned. We'll go for a walk along the river and watch the scullers in the late afternoon when the coming night air draws mist from the water. I like the end of the day, that enveloping pause between two worlds; just like Kurt used to stand on his back stoop drinking a beer at twilight and breathing in the city. Vera told me that in the long letter (book) she wrote me while she was institutionalized, after she killed my father. He didn't know about me. I was just a smattering of substances in Vera's belly when she pulled the trigger. Poor Kurt, mistaken for the man from Marrakesh who never, never was, or was he? That's what I don't know.

Vera's book is so convincing I get goose bumps when she describes "this speck of shadow trailing me across two continents." They never found him; they judged her mind, her imagination, guilty.

I never told James that Vera died of an overdose. It happens so easily in institutions, pills hidden, stored up, a dispensary door left unlocked, a sympathetic orderly. The report said she "expired" between early-morning rounds. It must have still been dark. I imagine she slipped away, scared at first, but then succumbing, like drowning. Maybe in her final moments my mother believed that the "evil chameleon" from Marrakesh would never catch her. She was free. They cremated her and for years her ashes were kept in an urn on a shelf in a storage closet. No one claimed them. They disappeared when the institution was renovated to take patients with insurance.

I won't tell James. This is my secret. I don't know if he ever knew anything about Vera after Kurt died. James went to live with his grandparents in Florida and then on to college and into the newspaper business. Maybe Vera wrote to him from the institution, the place where I was born and taken from before I even suckled, handed over for adoption. I doubt it. Vera only wrote that long letter-book to me, her daughter. That's what I like to think. But James and I were orphans, taken in by people who loved us, yes, but raised away from the magic of Kurt and Vera. It must have been magical; listening to James talk about the time on Virginia Beach with Vera laughing in her straw fedora and Kurt sleeping on the sand and getting burned and the waves crashing down and the Impala, with its top down, waiting to whisk them away like a flying carpet. I would have loved even a minute of that. I won't tell James he is my half brother, either. I've decided I could not bear his forgetting such a thing so cherished minutes after I uttered the words. I will keep it to myself. It is enough that I have found him and can check his blood pressure, sit with him by the window, and lay his clothes out in the morning. He's reading his old newspaper clippings. They don't register; all those lands and cities, all that joy and suffering he witnessed and wrote about mean nothing to him now.

Vera was a writer, too. On page sixty-seven in her letter-book she tells me: "Daughter, will I ever see you? I am trapped behind this wire and stone, and there is no way to you. Where would I look? I am good with maps, but maps need destinations and I don't know where they've taken you. But you are safe. A good couple loves you, this is what they tell me. They give me shreds of news from the world beyond, the world where you are growing up without me. I will write some more later. They're bringing my pills — yellow, blue, and white — and after I take them I get drowsy and I sit in a chair on the lawn and take my slippers off. The grass tickles my feet. Sometimes I think I see the man from Marrakesh, this Mounir, standing outside the iron fence in the shadows. But the people here tell me there is no one there, only tree branches moving in the wind. But that's what they would say, wouldn't they?"

James puts his newspaper clippings on the windowsill and stands and looks down the street. He is agitated; he gets this way, I think, when a memory flashes inside him and almost brings him back, but then leaves him. This is what doctors call Depletion. A terrible word. I hate to see it written in the charts, reducing someone to such a sad description. Science and medicine are cruel, but I suppose they must be. James turns from the window and sits on his bed. He stares at me as if I am a riddle.

"Do you know Kurt and Vera?" he says.

"Tell me about them."

"Where is Kurt buried?"

"Not far."

"Will you take me there?"

"Yes."

I help James into a sweater and a coat. I tie a scarlet scarf around him.

"It's cold. Do you want gloves?"

"No."

We walk outside and cross the street and take a right at the tailor's — an old Armenian man whose glasses have so magnified his eyes that they look like floating blue moons — and then we walk straight for seven blocks, and that's when James begins to know where he is.

"It's Clare Street. That's my old house."

"Someone else lives there now, James. You left many years ago."

"Yes, but this is it. Kurt boxed in the basement. He'd hit the punching bag so hard, the house shook."

"This way."

"That's St. Jude's. Kurt and I came here on Saturday nights. He played tennis on Sunday, so Saturday was our mass day."

James and I step through the church gate and walk over a sidewalk cracked by elm and chestnut roots. We haven't been here in a long time. The church is not well tended these days; most of the congregation moved to the suburbs and broken panes of stained glass have been replaced with colored cellophane. A boy — he's not here today; it's nearly winter — mows the cemetery grass and clips around the gravestones. The trees lend a sense of peace. James and I walk the rows toward Kurt. I hear a shuffle behind us.

"Jim Ryan?"

The priest is bent, white-haired; his clerical collar too wide for his thin neck. A dark coat hangs off him, and he balances on a cane, a bronze cross dangling over his chest. The cold makes his nose run, and he sniffs and pulls a handkerchief from his pocket, but with his unsteady hand the handkerchief dances before him like a puppet. He is frailer than when James and I last saw him, and I don't know why he is alone out here in this weather.

"Jim, it's me, Father Heaney."

James steps closer. He peers into Father's eyes. James hugs him and starts to weep.

"It is you."

"Not gone yet, Jim. Not gone yet, although some days I feel the Lord tugging fierce. I'm retired now, Jim. They gave me a room in the rectory, not the big one I used to have; that went to the new head honcho. I'm up near the attic in that little room we used to store stuff in."

Father laughs, looks to me, and dips his head. It has been a while, but he knows James is lost. I brought James here two years ago and explained his condition. Father said a prayer over him back then, made the sign of the cross and kissed him on the forehead and told him that the Lord would keep a light on inside James and one day James would find it. I'd stop in from time to time and visit Father, asking him about Kurt and James in the days before Vera. One afternoon, he was sweeping the vestibule when I came in and sat in a pew. He slid next to me and I told him that James was my brother and Kurt my father; he held my hand and as we stared at the white marble of the altar and up to the golden crucifix, I felt a burden lifted.

"You're here to see Kurt, huh, Jim?"

"Yes, Father. He and that time, the one summer, are the clearest things to me."

"I know, Jim."

Father's cane taps the broken sidewalk. I walk close behind him in case he stumbles. James is at his side. Kurt's resting place is the third one in from a tree, between Bobby Laughlin, a welder, and Chris O'Boyle, a rookie cop shot and killed one night on patrol. I still cry when I see Kurt's grave, and I'm crying now, looking at the gray stone, pretty calligraphy around its edges and a cross at its center, laid on this ground before I was born. James kneels and runs a finger across the shallow rivulets of Kurt's name and dates. He takes off his scarf and polishes in slow circles, a dull gleam rises through the grit. He stands and drapes the scarf over the stone.

"I always felt bad, Jim, that Kurt and your mother weren't buried side by side. Her family bought their plots years before she met Kurt. She lies over there, near the corner along the fence. You knew this once, but you may have forgotten. You visited her when you were a boy, before you moved away, and you'd sit over her for hours reading her words out of that dictionary of yours. You loved words. You used to try to disguise your sins in big words when you'd come to confession. I guess you thought they didn't sting as much that way."

"Do you still read mystery novels, Father?"

"I do."

Kids walking home from school hurry past the cemetery. Little tilted armies with book bags dangling. James looks toward them and back to the brown grass beneath his feet. The sky feels like snow.

"The day before Kurt died we swam in the ocean beyond where the waves begin to lift and curl. The water is calm out there, Father. We floated and talked. The tide moved deep beneath us. We could see specks of people on the beach, but we couldn't hear them. Even the seagulls were silent. Kurt told me about the ships he painted and how far they sailed, and he told me to make sure I see the world because he said he wondered what it would be like to be standing on one of those ships as it sailed into a faraway port."

"You saw a lot of the world, Jim."

James steps back from the grave. Father holds his one hand. I hold his other. We stand in silence. Lights click on in nearby row houses, silhouettes in windows, dinners on stoves, homework undone. The factory and dock men will be heading home soon, walking through alleys beneath sputtering streetlights, opening doors and listening to voices that will carry them toward sleep. There is peace in the twilight. James's scarf blows off Kurt's marker and tumbles across the dead. The scarlet is pretty against the gray. The scarf lifts in the wind, twirling like a bird or a bright rag toward the coming moon.

ACKNOWLEDGMENTS

Shadow Man would not have been possible without Sorche Fairbank, my agent, and Chip Fleischer and Roland Pease at Steerforth Press. I thank Peter Holm at Sterling Hill Productions and Kari Howard at the *Los Angeles Times* for her style and grace with words. A special gratitude goes to Marcella Aigner and Angie Slattery for the wisdom in the stories they have told. And, as ever, my thanks to Clare, Aaron and Hannah.

Jeffrey Fleishman is the Cairo bureau chief for the *Los Angeles Times*. A Pulitzer Prize finalist and former Nieman Fellow at Harvard University, he has covered the revolutions of Arab Spring and wars in Kosovo, Iraq and Libya. He is the author of *Promised Virgins: A Novel of Jihad*.

Reading Group Guide for
SHADOW MAN
by Jeffrey Fleishman

Note: Before your group begins discussing *Shadow Man*, invite each member to take one minute to present his or her general impression of the book, without interruption or comments from the other members. This preamble to group discussion provides an opportunity for everyone to voice their opinion, and does not hinder the discussion that follows.

QUESTIONS FOR DISCUSSION

1. Describe the relationship between Jim and Kurt.

2. Discuss the narrative points when Vera went from enchanting story-teller to dangerously delusional.

3. What role does Jim's dead mother play?

4. What does Jim's journey with Kurt and Vera to Virginia Beach symbolize?

5. How does the relationship between Kurt and Vera affect Jim, if indeed it does?

6. The lady in white hovers at the edge of James' recollections. What kept her so composed?

7. What do you think of the depiction of early onset Alzheimer's from James' point of view? Is this how you you would imagine it to be?

8. Discuss the bonds that held Eva and James together as they chased newspaper stories across the world. Does anything remain of those original bonds?

9. When Eva left James in the next to last chapter, did you think that she would ever return?

10. What part does Alice play in the coming-of-age narrative that is Jim's only remaining memory?

11. Was there ever a man from Marrakesh, and if so, how much of Vera's story seems to be true?

12. Are we the sum of our memories, and what happens to us when they're gone?

13. What are the similarities and contrasts between the central female characters - Vera, Eva and the lady in white?

14. Was the novel redemptive, or in the end were James and those who loved him doomed to a single memory?